EAST RENFREWSHIRE COUNCIL

0803915 1

24 APR 2008

31 JL

D0532631

03 OCT 1

JULY 2012

-3 JUN 2009

02 NOV 2009

15 MAY 2013

27 DEC 2018

-5 MAR 2010

29 JUL 2010

-9 SEP 2010

22 AUG 2011

15 NOV 2011

Return this item by
the last date shown.

Items may be renewed
by telephone or at
www.eastrenfrewshire.gov.uk/libraries

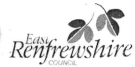

East
Renfrewshire
COUNCIL

IMPORTANT NOTICE
This book is intended not as a substitute for personal
medical advice but as a supplement to that advice for
the patient who wishes to understand more about his or
her condition.

Before taking any form of treatment
YOU SHOULD ALWAYS CONSULT YOUR MEDICAL
PRACTITIONER.

In particular (without limit) you should note that
advances in medical science occur rapidly and some
information about drugs and treatment contained in this
booklet may very soon be out of date.

All rights reserved. No part of this publication may be reproduced, or
stored in a retrieval system, or transmitted, in any form or by any means,
electronic, mechanical, photocopying, recording and/or otherwise,
without the prior written permission of the publishers. The right of Dr
Joan Webster-Gandy to be identified as the author of this work has been
asserted in accordance with the Copyright, Designs and Patents Act
1988, Sections 77 and 78.

EAST RENFREWSHIRE COUNCIL	
08039151	
HJ	07/02/2008
613.2	£4.75

© Family Doctor Publications 2002–2006
Updated 2002, 2004, 2006

Family Doctor Publications, PO Box 4664, Poole, Dorset BH15 1NN

ISBN: 1 903474 41 8

Contents

About the author

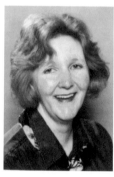

Dr Joan Webster-Gandy is Reader in Nutrition at Buckingham Chilterns University College, a State Registered Dietitian and a Registered Nutritionist with the Nutrition Society. Her research interests include obesity and related diseases. She has a wide experience of dietetics and public health nutrition.

Introduction

The importance of food

The food that you eat has a strong influence on your health and on your chances of developing diseases including heart disease and some types of cancer. This book is aimed at people who are basically healthy, to help them understand nutrition and choose a diet that will keep them in good health.

The opening chapters explain in detail how you digest food and why your body needs:

- energy

- protein

- fat

- carbohydrates

- vitamins and minerals.

These chapters include the science of nutrition, good food sources and links with illnesses, such as heart and bowel diseases and cancer.

Healthy eating

The chapter 'Healthy eating' enables you to put the information together so that you can plan a diet that incorporates appropriate amounts of the various food groups. This chapter also includes information on the safest and most effective way to lose weight.

To make informed choices about your diet, you need to know how to read the nutritional labelling on food packets, and to be aware of the various ways in which fresh produce may have been treated to increase its acceptability to consumers. This is covered in the chapters 'Food labelling' and 'Food additives'.

Some people can't eat certain foods or food additives for health reasons, even foods that are essential to a balanced diet. The chapter 'Food allergy and intolerance' gives information and advice about this.

There are many different nutritional products and diets available, which are claimed to enhance a balanced diet or to encourage rapid weight loss. These are discussed in the final chapter 'Dietary supplements, alternative diets and "health foods"'.

This book provides an overview of nutrition. For people requiring further information on specific medical conditions or nutritional requirements (for example, vegans), there is a list of useful addresses at the back of the book (see page 126).

KEY POINT

- The food that you eat has a strong influence on your health and on your chances of developing heart disease and some types of cancer

How your body uses food

Turning food into nutrients

Everything that goes into your stomach is mixed with enzymes, chemicals that break food down into its basic components (nutrients). The mixture is then passed from your stomach into your intestines, where the nutrients are absorbed into your bloodstream. Your blood transports the nutrients around your body to the cells where they are used or stored. Food components that are not absorbed are excreted.

Your gastrointestinal tract

Your gastrointestinal tract is a tube around seven metres long, which begins at your mouth and ends at your anus. Each section of the tube has its role to play in digestion.

The mouth

Digestion begins as soon as you start chewing food. Saliva, secreted by glands in your mouth, is mixed with the food as you chew it, to make it easier to swallow.

Saliva contains an enzyme called amylase, which

The gastrointestinal tract

Digestion starts in the mouth and continues in the stomach and small intestine. Nutrients are absorbed in the intestines and waste materials are excreted through the anus.

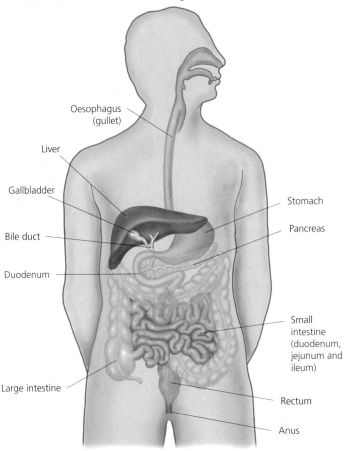

Oesophagus (gullet)

Liver

Gallbladder

Bile duct

Duodenum

Large intestine

Stomach

Pancreas

Small intestine (duodenum, jejunum and ileum)

Rectum

Anus

breaks down starchy carbohydrate foods into simpler sugars that can be absorbed into your body. Amylase can work only in an alkaline environment, such as in the mouth.

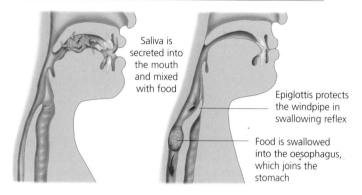

Saliva is secreted into the mouth and mixed with food

Epiglottis protects the windpipe in swallowing reflex

Food is swallowed into the oesophagus, which joins the stomach

Saliva is mixed with food as you chew, making it easier to swallow and starting digestion.

The stomach

Once food is swallowed, it travels down your oesophagus (gullet) to your stomach. At its entrance and exit, your stomach has rings of muscle called sphincters, which act as valves. When food arrives at your stomach, the top sphincter opens so that food can enter. The top sphincter then closes, keeping the food and digestive juices inside your stomach. If this sphincter leaks, digestive juices, including acid, are regurgitated into your gullet. When this happens, you experience heartburn, as your stomach's acid contents irritate the lining of your oesophagus.

Digestive juices are added to food from glands in your stomach wall. These juices contain chemicals that break down food into a usable form. Two of the chemicals are the enzyme protease and hydrochloric acid. Protease breaks down proteins. Hydrochloric acid destroys most of the bacteria present in food and provides the acid conditions in which protease works.

Only one substance is not subject to these digestive processes: alcohol is absorbed into your bloodstream directly from your stomach.

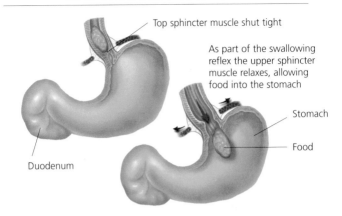

Top sphincter muscle shut tight

As part of the swallowing reflex the upper sphincter muscle relaxes, allowing food into the stomach

Stomach

Food

Duodenum

The stomach has rings of muscle at its entrance and exit, which act as valves, sealing the stomach.

Your stomach acts as a reservoir. Semi-liquid food remains there for two to four hours before being released in small amounts, through the lower sphincter, into your small intestine.

The small intestine

This is the longest part of your gastrointestinal tract, being five to six metres long. It is called the 'small' intestine because it is narrow, only two to four centimetres in diameter, compared with the large intestine, which is six centimetres in diameter.

Your small intestine has three distinct parts:

1 the duodenum, which lies just after your stomach, and is the shortest part of your small intestine

2 the jejunum

3 the ileum, which connects to your large intestine.

When food enters your duodenum, it is still acid from the stomach juices. Alkaline digestive juices are now added to neutralise it. They are produced in the

The digestive process

Food passes from the stomach into the small intestine, where absorption of nutrients begins. The large intestine comes after the small intestine. It absorbs water and eliminates undigested waste.

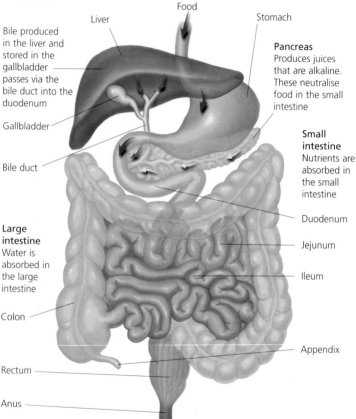

Food

Liver

Stomach

Bile produced in the liver and stored in the gallbladder passes via the bile duct into the duodenum

Pancreas
Produces juices that are alkaline. These neutralise food in the small intestine

Gallbladder

Small intestine
Nutrients are absorbed in the small intestine

Bile duct

Duodenum

Large intestine
Water is absorbed in the large intestine

Jejunum

Ileum

Colon

Appendix

Rectum

Anus

pancreas, just below your stomach, and they contain enzymes that continue to digest food. Bile is also added to the mixture. This green, watery fluid, which is produced in your liver and stored in your gallbladder, helps to keep fatty material in solution.

Villi of the small intestine

The intestinal wall is not smooth but consists of millions of tiny finger-like protrusions called villi.

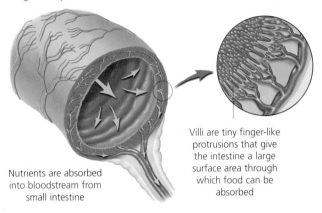

Nutrients are absorbed into bloodstream from small intestine

Villi are tiny finger-like protrusions that give the intestine a large surface area through which food can be absorbed

Once the digestive juices have done their job, the major food components have been broken down into their constituents:

- proteins into amino acids

- carbohydrates into glucose and other simple sugars

- fat into fatty acids and glycerol.

The jejunum and ileum

Further down your small intestine, in your jejunum and ileum, the end-products of digestion are absorbed through the intestinal wall into your bloodstream. Food is passed along your intestine by wave-like contractions of muscles in the intestinal wall; this is called peristalsis. The intestinal wall is not smooth, but consists of millions of tiny finger-like protrusions called villi. The villi give your intestines a large surface area through which food is absorbed. Water-soluble vitamins and minerals are also absorbed at this stage of digestion.

Once the nutrients have been absorbed, the remaining undigested food passes through another sphincter muscle into your large intestine. Your body can store some nutrients, such as those providing energy and certain vitamins and minerals. Excesses of nutrients that cannot be stored are lost in the faeces.

The large intestine

Your large intestine consists of your colon, rectum and anus, and is up to one metre in length. It reabsorbs the water that is used in digestion and eliminates undigested food and fibre. It has recently been shown that very little food is really passed through the body undigested, because bacteria in the colon break down fibre residues, and release fatty acids, which are important for the nutrition of the colon itself. Once water has been reabsorbed in your colon, the faeces, which are now drier and more solid, are passed along your rectum by peristalsis and are finally expelled through your anus.

When faeces reach your rectum, they trigger the desire to defecate, owing to reflex contractions of your rectum and the relaxation of your anal sphincter muscles. Your anal sphincters are circular muscles that control the opening and closing of your anus.

It usually takes between one and three days for food to pass from your mouth to your anus. Some people defecate two or three times a day, others daily and some only every two to three days. All of these patterns are normal.

The importance of fibre

Fibre or non-starch polysaccharides (NSPs) are derived from plant material. Fibre cannot be broken down by digestive enzymes, so it passes through your gastrointestinal tract without being absorbed. As it

Fibre and regular bowel movements

If you eat a high-fibre diet with plenty of fluids, your faeces will be bulky. This stimulates the gut wall, increasing peristalsis and preventing constipation.

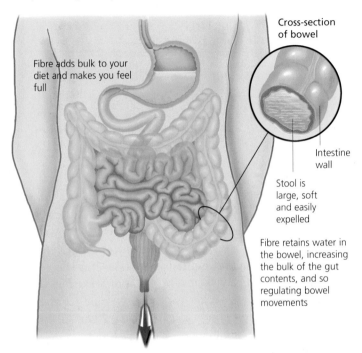

Cross-section of bowel

Fibre adds bulk to your diet and makes you feel full

Intestine wall

Stool is large, soft and easily expelled

Fibre retains water in the bowel, increasing the bulk of the gut contents, and so regulating bowel movements

adds bulk to your diet, fibre makes you feel full and also regulates your bowel movements. It does this by retaining water in your gut, increasing the bulk of the gut contents.

Constipation

If you eat a high-fibre diet with plenty of fluids, your faeces will be bulky. As a result, they stimulate your gut wall, increasing peristalsis, and pass through more quickly and easily. This prevents constipation, which affects 10 to 12 per cent of the population. This figure

Diverticular disease

Straining to pass hard faeces can stretch the wall of the large intestine, forming small pouches called diverticula.

Normal colon   **Colon with diverticula**

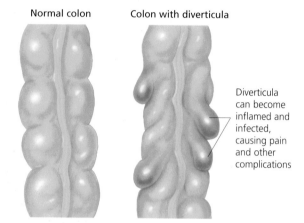

Diverticula can become inflamed and infected, causing pain and other complications

rises to 20 to 30 per cent of those aged over 60.

Some people think that they have constipation simply because they don't realise that their bowel habits are actually normal. Changing to a high-fibre diet and drinking more fluids can ease constipation in most people. Laxatives should be used only on medical advice, as they are not always necessary and their abuse can lead to other problems, such as loss of muscle tone in the bowel.

Diverticular disease

A high-fibre diet also helps prevent a common disorder called diverticular disease. The early stages of this can be detected in at least 15 per cent of people over 50. Most sufferers have a history of constipation, which leads to increased pressure in the colon. Straining to pass hard faeces can stretch the wall of the large intestine, encouraging the formation of small pouches, called diverticula, which are pushed outwards from the bowel wall. Inflammation and bacterial overgrowth in these pouches may cause pain and diarrhoea. A high-fibre diet with plenty of fluids can relieve the symptoms in most people. Some people, however, will require treatment with laxatives.

Bowel cancer

Fibre in the diet is also important in connection with bowel cancer, the third most common type of cancer. If detected early enough, it has a very good prognosis, but many people delay seeking medical advice because of embarrassment. It has been shown that a diet that is low in fibre increases the risk of developing bowel cancer. This is because, without fibre, unabsorbed food takes longer to pass through the gut. This means that the bowel lining is exposed to potentially harmful compounds in the unabsorbed food for longer periods.

Case study: diverticular disease

Tom, a widower in his 70s, had suffered from intermittent diarrhoea and severe pains in his lower abdomen for a couple of weeks. When his doctor questioned him about his bowel habits, it became clear that Tom frequently suffered from constipation. Analysis of his faeces showed that Tom didn't have an infection. A barium enema, which gives a picture of the lining of the large intestine, showed that Tom was suffering from diverticular disease. He was referred to a dietitian, who discovered that Tom's diet didn't include much fibre and that he drank only small amounts of fluid. She advised Tom on how to increase the amount of fibre in his diet while still enjoying his favourite foods. She also encouraged him to increase his fluid intake. By following this advice, Tom was able to relieve many of his symptoms.

KEY POINTS

- Food is broken down into its building blocks by enzymes in your mouth, stomach and small intestine

- Nutrients are absorbed into your bloodstream from your intestine

- Some excess nutrients can be stored in your body, but others are excreted

- Fibre is essential for the normal movement of food along your bowel and has a key role in food digestion and absorption

Energy

Calories

Your body's primary need, apart from water, is for energy. When your body needs energy, you feel hungry. The amount of energy that you need and use is measured in calories.

A thousand calories make up a kilocalorie (kcal) or Calorie (with a capital C). In ordinary speech, when people use the word 'calories', they actually mean kilocalories. This book also uses the word 'calories' (with a small c), in that everyday way, to refer to kilocalories.

Energy may also be measured in joules or thousands of joules (kilojoules or kJ): 1 kcal = 4.2 kJ.

Calories are often used as a negative term, with people worrying about taking in too many. In contrast, people talk positively about having 'lots of energy', meaning that they feel healthy. In nutritional terms, however, calories and energy are the same thing.

Why you need energy

Your body needs energy for life, voluntary activities (such as movement) and special purposes such as pregnancy, breast-feeding and growth. You need it to breathe, digest and absorb food and maintain your body temperature.

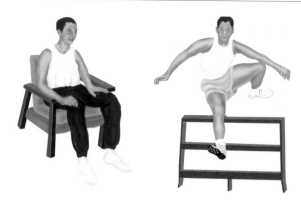

Any activity, no matter how small (even sitting up), uses energy. The more activity you do, the more calories you burn up.

The rate at which you use energy is known as your metabolic rate. Your resting metabolic rate (RMR) is the number of kilocalories or kilojoules that you use just by existing (breathing, pumping blood around your body, etc.) and represents about 70 per cent of your total energy expenditure.

How much energy do you need?

The chart on page 17 shows the amount of energy needed by men and women of average weights, with sedentary occupations, who don't do much exercise. If your level of activity increases, either at work or because you start to take more exercise, your total energy requirement will increase too.

Your energy requirements change at different stages of your life, for example growth requires a lot of energy. A child uses up less energy than an adult. However, if you compare energy requirements per kilogram of body weight, a child actually uses up a higher proportion of energy per body weight than an adult.

Approximate energy expenditure

All activities burn calories. However, the more strenuous the activity that you undertake, the more calories you burn and the greater your total energy requirement.

Activity	kcal per minute	kJ per minute
Sitting	1.4	6
Walking slowly	3	13
Golf	2.5–4.9	10–20
Housework	2.5–4.9	10–20
Digging	5.0–7.4	21–30
Playing squash	7.5+	32+
Aerobic exercise	7–9	29–38

After maturity, the adult energy requirement is fairly constant, but shows a slight, and continuing, decline from the age of 30.

Energy requirements increase during pregnancy to meet the needs of the uterus, placenta and fetus. A pregnant woman's blood volume increases and she lays down extra fatty tissue. The increase in estimated average requirement (EAR) for pregnancy in the last trimester, from around week 26, is 200 kcal per day.

A woman who is breast-feeding needs, on average, an extra 500 kcal per day to maintain a good supply of milk.

Why men need more energy than women

Your body weight is determined by two components: fat and fat-free mass (FFM). Fat-free mass consists of your body's lean tissues, including muscle, bone, blood

Estimated average requirements of energy needed for men and women of average weight and in sedentary occupations

Age	kcal per day	MJ per day (1,000 kJ = 1 MJ)
Males		
0–3 months	545	2.28
4–6 months	690	2.89
7–9 months	825	3.44
10–12 months	920	3.85
1–3 years	1,230	5.15
4–6 years	1,715	7.16
7–10 years	1,970	8.24
11–14 years	2,220	9.27
15–18 years	2,755	11.51
19–50 years	2,550	10.60
51–59 years	2,550	10.60
60–64 years	2,380	9.93
65–74 years	2,330	9.71
75+ years	2,100	8.77
Females		
0–3 months	515	2.16
4–6 months	645	2.69
7–9 months	765	3.20
10–12 months	865	3.61
1–3 years	1,165	4.86
4–6 years	1,545	6.46
7–10 years	1,740	7.28
11–14 years	1,845	7.92
15–18 years	2,110	8.83
19–50 years	1,940	8.10
51–59 years	1,900	8.00
60–64 years	1,900	7.99
65–74 years	1,900	7.96
75+ years	1,810	7.61
Pregnancy – additional requirement		
(6–9 months)	+200	+0.80
Lactation	+450–480	+1.9–2.0

and internal organs. These structures are responsible for most of your energy consumption. The amount of FFM you have determines how many calories you use, as fat itself burns very few calories. Men have a higher proportion of FFM than women and therefore burn more calories. This means that a man needs more calories per day than a woman of the same age and weight.

Gaining and losing weight

If you eat the same amount of calories as you use up, your weight will remain constant. If you eat more calories than you need, your weight will increase. To lose weight, you need to use more calories than you take in.

Over a long period, any excess energy is stored as fat. If your energy intake exceeds your energy output by 7,000 kcal, you will gain 1 kilogram (2.2 pounds) in weight. It doesn't matter if you eat these extra calories in one sitting or over a period of days or weeks, the weight gain will be the same, although the rate of weight gain will differ.

The additional weight will not be pure fat, but 75 per cent fat and 25 per cent FFM (fat-free mass). This is because extra lean tissue (for example, cell walls, blood vessels and connective tissue) is needed to support the extra fat. The increased amount of FFM in your body will mean that you need more energy.

If you continue to eat more than you need, you will continue to gain weight. To lose weight, you must eat fewer calories. As you lose weight, you lose FFM and lower your energy requirements. This means that you will need to take in even less energy if you are to continue losing weight. When you reach your target weight, you can consume the amount of calories that will balance your energy intake with your energy expenditure and you will then stabilise at your new weight.

For more on weight loss, see 'Healthy eating' on page 75.

Where does energy come from?

Energy in your diet is provided by carbohydrate, fat, protein and alcohol. Almost all the weight of a food is made up of these components plus water. Some foods, such as many

Energy values

The following table gives the energy or calorific values of carbohydrate, fat, protein, alcohol and water – the basic food components.

Nutrient	kcal per gram	kJ per gram
Carbohydrate	4	17
Fat	9	38
Protein	4	17
Alcohol	7	29
Water	0	0

The following foods all contain approximately 100 kcal

- 150 ml (half a mug) whole milk
- 290 ml (one mug) skimmed milk
- 290 ml (approx. half a pint) lager
- 2 slices wholemeal bread
- 25 g Cheddar cheese
- 20 g chocolate
- 95 g potato baked in jacket
- 1 kg cooked cauliflower
- A third (approx.) of a Mars bar
- 50 g bag of crisps

fruit and vegetables, contain a lot of water, which has no calorific value, and have less protein, fat or carbohydrate for a given weight and are therefore low in calories.

A fatty food, such as butter, which contains relatively little water, is rich in calories. The energy or calorific value of the food components is given in the table on page 20.

Alcohol

Alcohol is a source of energy but contains no other nutrients. It is rapidly absorbed from your stomach and slowly broken down (metabolised) by your liver. The rate at which this occurs determines how quickly you become intoxicated.

The rate of metabolism varies from one person to another and depends on their size. Generally, smaller people metabolise alcohol more slowly than large

What is a unit of alcohol?

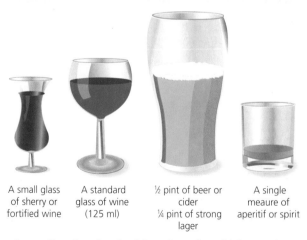

A small glass of sherry or fortified wine

A standard glass of wine (125 ml)

½ pint of beer or cider ¼ pint of strong lager

A single meaure of aperitif or spirit

A one-litre bottle of spirits – brandy, whisky or gin – contains about 40 units of alcohol

people, and women more slowly than men. Drinking alcohol with food slows down the rate at which the alcohol is absorbed from your stomach, so that it has a less intoxicating effect.

The maximum recommended intake of alcohol is three units a day for men and two units a day for women. Two days per week should be alcohol free. A unit provides about eight grams of alcohol and is equivalent to one small glass of wine, half a pint of beer or one pub measure of spirits. Drinking more than the recommended amount increases the social and physical hazards.

Recent studies have shown a relationship between moderate intakes of alcohol and a decrease in the rate of coronary heart disease. The mechanism for this is unclear, although it is thought that alcohol probably has a beneficial effect on certain types of fat in the bloodstream that help to stop the arteries becoming clogged.

KEY POINTS

- Your body needs energy to survive

- Children have higher energy requirements than adults in relation to their body weight; older people have lower energy requirements

- Fat is your body's main energy store and is used when you don't eat enough food

- People put on weight when their energy intake exceeds their energy requirements

Protein

Proteins in your body

Proteins are the building blocks of your body. Without them, you would not be able to replace or repair your body cells. An average 70-kilogram man contains about 11 kilograms of protein. Nearly half of this is found in skeletal muscle.

Why you need protein

Protein has many important uses in your body. It is a major component of structural tissues such as skin and collagen, which is found in connective tissue such as tendons and ligaments. Blood requires protein for red blood cells, white blood cells and numerous compounds in plasma. Your body's immunity is also dependent on protein, which is needed for the formation of antibodies and white blood cells that fight disease. Enzymes and some hormones (for example, insulin) are also proteins.

If your diet doesn't provide enough energy, your body will eventually use functional body proteins (proteins that are incorporated into the essential structure of your body). Your body can adapt to a lack of protein in the short term. However, conditions such as injury, infection, cancer, uncontrolled diabetes and starvation can cause substantial protein losses. In these circumstances, the body starts to lose muscle in order to generate enough energy. If left unchecked, this can become life threatening.

What are proteins?

Proteins are large compounds of smaller units called amino acids. Amino acids contain carbon, hydrogen, oxygen, nitrogen and occasionally sulphur. All amino acids have an acid group and an amino group attached to different carbon atoms. 'Amino' is the chemical name for the combination of nitrogen and hydrogen in these compounds.

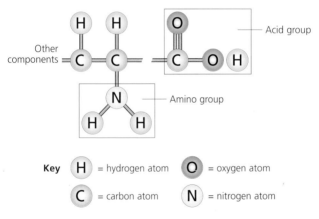

This diagram shows the chemical structure of an amino acid.

The amino group of one amino acid can link with the acid group of another amino acid to form a dipeptide. The link is called a peptide bond. When more than two amino acids join together, a polypeptide is formed. A typical protein may contain 500 or more amino acids joined together.

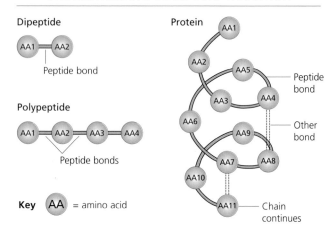

Amino acids join together by peptide bonds to form polypeptides, which can be complex chains. Their size and shape determine what protein is formed and its function.

The size and shape of each polypeptide determine what protein it is and its function. Some proteins are made of several polypeptides. Each species has its own characteristic proteins. The proteins of human muscle, for instance, are different from those of beef muscle.

How your body uses proteins

Proteins are broken down into amino acids and small peptides by enzymes (proteases) in your gut. The small peptides and amino acids are taken via your bloodstream to your liver, where they are used or transported to your body's cells.

Your liver is the most important site of amino acid and protein metabolism. Amino acids are chemically changed so that they can be used for energy, or converted into other amino acids or proteins, or into urea (the form in which they are excreted). Some proteins, such as collagen in connective tissue or

The metabolism of protein

Proteins are broken down by enzymes in the small intestine. The digested components are then transported in the bloodstream to the liver to be metabolised.

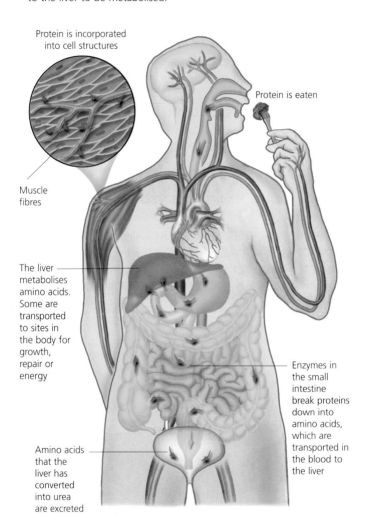

Protein is incorporated into cell structures

Protein is eaten

Muscle fibres

The liver metabolises amino acids. Some are transported to sites in the body for growth, repair or energy

Enzymes in the small intestine break proteins down into amino acids, which are transported in the blood to the liver

Amino acids that the liver has converted into urea are excreted

tendons, are very resistant to digestion and pass through your gut unchanged to be excreted.

All the proteins that your body needs can be made from 20 different amino acids. You can make some of these from other amino acids, but there are eight that can't be made by your body and must be supplied by your diet. These are called essential amino acids. Children need a further two amino acids for growth.

Where is protein found?

Protein can be found in animal produce such as meat, fish, eggs, milk and milk products, and in plant foods such as cereals, beans and pulses. All protein sources contain some of the essential amino acids but in varying amounts. Some foods, such as milk and eggs, contain almost the ideal mixture of amino acids, but usually miss out one essential amino acid or contain it in small, inadequate amounts. It is therefore important to eat a mixture of protein sources to ensure that you have an adequate supply of all the essential amino acids.

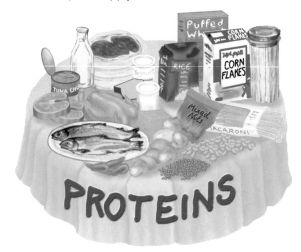

How much protein do you need?

The staple foods that make up the average diet in the UK have a fairly high ratio of protein to energy. It is very unlikely that a person whose diet provides enough energy will be deficient in protein. However, this may happen if their diet contains a lot of 'empty calories', such as sugar or alcohol, which provide energy but little protein.

Protein requirements

The recommended amount of protein in your daily diet is determined primarily by your age and sex. The figures set out in the table below are the estimated average requirements (EARs).

Children 0–10	g/day
< 1 year	11.0
1–3 years	11.7
4–6 years	14.8
7–10 years	22.8

Males from age 11	
11–14 years	33.8
15–18 years	46.1
19–50 years	44.4
50+ years	42.6

Females from age 11	
11–14 years	33.1
15–18 years	37.1
19–50 years	36.0
50+ years	37.2

The WHO (World Health Organization) does not give figures for 0–3 months, so no EAR can be derived. To save confusion, all babies < 1 year have been put together.

Examples of foods containing approximately six grams of protein

- Milk (whole)   200 ml
- Egg   1 medium/size 3
- Baked beans   6 tablespoons
- Red meat   20 grams
- Chicken   25 grams
- Cheese   25 grams
- Pasta   50 grams

Special needs

Children, vegetarians, vegans and pregnant or breast-feeding women need to ensure that they have enough protein in their diet.

Children

Children need extra protein so that they can grow properly. The estimated average requirement (EAR) of a four- to six-month-old baby is more than twice that of an adult, at 1.4 grams per kilogram of body weight per day. It is estimated that more than 40 per cent of an infant's protein intake should be essential amino acids. The mixture of essential amino acids should be in the correct proportions. This falls to 32 per cent in pre-school children and 22 per cent in 10 to 12 year olds. Adults need 11 per cent.

As already stated, there are two extra essential amino acids that children need for growth. These are found in the same protein sources as the other essential amino acids. Vegan or macrobiotic diets, which contain no animal produce (including dairy products), are not suitable for small children. They are unlikely to provide all the essential amino acids. As they contain large amounts of bulky fibrous foods, these diets are unlikely to supply sufficient energy as fat or carbohydrate and, therefore, protein may be used to make up the deficit.

Vegetarians and vegans

Provided that you follow guidelines on what constitutes a balanced diet, you can get all the essential amino acids and other nutrients that you need without eating meat or fish. However, you should mix your sources of protein. Dietary guidelines vary, depending on what types of food you choose to avoid. An ova-lacto-vegetarian eats animal proteins such as eggs, milk and milk products, especially cheese. A vegan who consumes only vegetable sources of protein may find it harder to ensure that they get all the necessary nutrients, but it certainly isn't impossible. It is advisable to make sure that you know how to balance your diet properly before becoming a vegan. There are various books available and the Vegan Society produces information and product lists.

If you are bringing up your child as a vegetarian, it is important to make sure that his or her energy needs are met. Weaning foods such as pulses, cereals, bananas and avocado pears should be given frequently. The timing of the introduction of some foods should follow current guidelines, for example wheat should not be introduced before one year of age. Aim to include two different plant sources of protein at each meal because this will provide a better balance of amino acids. It will probably be necessary to supplement your child's diet with vitamins and minerals. This should ideally be done in consultation with health professionals, such as a health visitor or dietitian.

Pregnant and breast-feeding women

A pregnant woman needs an extra six grams of pure protein daily to allow her baby to grow and develop properly. This will also meet her own needs, which increase as she develops extra body tissues.

Breast-feeding is very demanding in terms of both energy and protein. To maintain an adequate milk supply, which is a rich source of protein, it is estimated that the mother requires an extra 11 grams of protein per day from birth until her baby is six months old. After this she needs eight grams extra per day. Most babies start eating some solids around this age.

If you are on a strict vegan or macrobiotic diet, you may need iron and vitamin supplements while pregnant or breast-feeding. Babies should not routinely be given soya milk because it is not supplemented with the necessary vitamins and minerals. You should discuss your diet and that of your baby with a qualified dietitian.

Case study: anaemia

Polly was born at full term and weighed 5 lb 8 oz (2.5 kg). Her mother Sue follows a macrobiotic diet and would like to bring up Polly to eat the same way. Sue breast-fed Polly and introduced solids when she reached five months. Polly began to sleep poorly, and her weight did not increase appreciably from the time she started on solids.

Sue's health visitor arranged a referral to the paediatrician at the local hospital. Investigations showed that Polly was anaemic and deficient in iron and vitamin B_{12}. It is likely that, as a result of her diet, Sue's breast milk was lacking in both these nutrients. The paediatric dietitian was able to advise Sue on how to wean Polly and maintain adequate nutrition while sticking to a vegetarian diet. She emphasised that strict macrobiotic diets are not suitable for children under two years of age.

KEY POINTS

- Proteins are made of amino acids

- Essential amino acids cannot be made in your body and therefore need to be obtained from food

- Vegetarian diets can be suitable for all age groups, but vegan diets are not suitable for children, especially those under school age

Fats

Visible and invisible fats

Fats (or lipids) in your diet are often divided into two
types: visible and invisible. Visible fats are those that are
obvious, such as butter, margarine and other spreads,
cooking oils and fat on meat. Invisible (hidden) fats are
incorporated during cooking (for example, in cakes and
biscuits) or during food preparation (as in sausages).
Emulsions of fat are used extensively in products such as
mayonnaise. Some foods such as eggs are also rich in fat.

Why do you need fat?

A great deal has been written about the harmful
effects of fat, but fat is an essential part of your diet
for three important reasons.

Taste

Fat makes many foods taste better. It's no use a food
being nutritious if people don't like it and therefore
won't eat it!

Energy

Fats are a concentrated source of energy, providing
nine kcal per gram (38 kJ per gram).

The structure of fatty acids

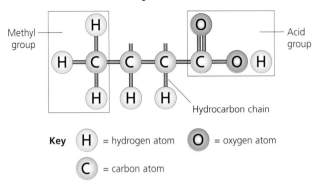

Methyl group

Acid group

Hydrocarbon chain

Key (H) = hydrogen atom (O) = oxygen atom

(C) = carbon atom

Essential nutrients
Fat in your diet provides fat-soluble vitamins (for more details, see 'Vitamins and minerals' on page 62) and essential fatty acids.

What are fats?

The basic building blocks of fat are fatty acids and glycerol. A fatty acid is made up of a chain of carbon atoms with an acid group at one end and a methyl group at the other. A methyl group consists of one carbon atom and three hydrogens.

Three different fatty acids combine with glycerol to form a triglyceride. The fat in your food is made up of a mixture of triglycerides.

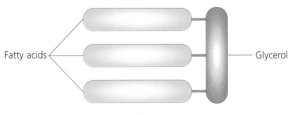

Fatty acids

Glycerol

Triglyceride.

Saturated and unsaturated fatty acids

If each carbon atom in the chain that makes up a fatty acid is attached to two hydrogen atoms, the fatty acid is said to be saturated. If hydrogen atoms are missing, it is said to be unsaturated.

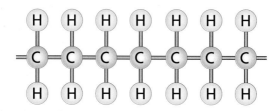

A saturated hydrocarbon chain, for example butter.

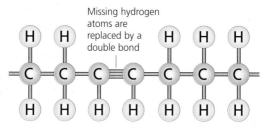

A monounsaturated hydrocarbon chain, for example olive oil.

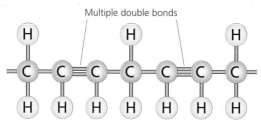

A polyunsaturated hydrocarbon chain, for example sunflower oil.

Key (H) = hydrogen atom (C) = carbon atom

Saturated and unsaturated fats

The amount and type of the fatty acids that you eat influence the way in which your body handles them and therefore their role in diseases such as coronary heart disease. Each carbon atom in a fatty acid chain is attached to one or two hydrogen atoms. If the fatty acid has all the hydrogen atoms that it can hold, it is said to be saturated.

If, however, some hydrogen atoms are missing, the fatty acid is said to be unsaturated. In unsaturated fats, the missing hydrogen atoms are replaced by a double bond between the carbon atoms.

All fats contain both saturated and unsaturated fatty acids, and the relative proportions of saturates and unsaturates give each fat its predominant characteristics (for example, oil or solid). The level of saturation of a fat is also referred to as hydrogenation. It is possible to alter this level of saturation (or hydrogenation) in the manufacture of fats and oils.

Generally, fats from animal sources, such as butter, have a high level of saturation. Saturated fats are more solid at room temperature than unsaturated fats.

Unsaturated fats are derived from vegetable sources. Monounsaturated fats have two hydrogen atoms missing from the fatty acid complex and therefore have one double bond.

Polyunsaturated fatty acids have more than two hydrogen atoms missing and, therefore, have more than one double bond.

The less saturated the fat molecule, the more liquid it will be. There are exceptions to this, such as coconut oil, which is a saturated fat but is liquid. Food manufacturers have developed ways of producing unsaturated solid fats by using stabilisers and emulsifiers. When margarine was first developed in France in 1869, it was made of animal fats and was therefore a saturated fat, but today it is made from vegetable oils and chemically hardened.

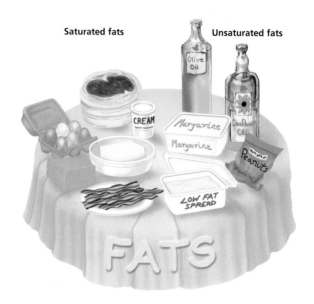

Saturated fats

Unsaturated fats

Fat is an essential part of the diet. Fats come from both animal and plant sources.

Essential fatty acids

Most fatty acids can be made in your body. However, linoleic acid and linolenic acid must be supplied by your diet. These are known as essential fatty acids (EFAs). Some others can be produced to a limited extent from these two essential fatty acids.

Essential fatty acids keep cell walls in good condition and working properly. They are also important in the transport, breakdown and excretion of cholesterol. They are used to manufacture other chemicals in your body such as prostaglandins. Dietary EFAs may also be involved in the brain development of babies. Most vegetable oils and oily fish are good sources of EFAs.

Examples of the varying proportions of the different kinds of fat in common foods

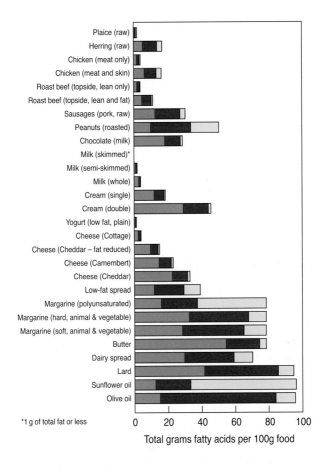

Total grams fatty acids per 100g food

*1 g of total fat or less

Key

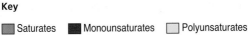

Saturates   Monounsaturates   Polyunsaturates

Omega 3 fatty acids

These fatty acids are found in oily fish and fish oils. An increase in their consumption has health benefits such as reducing the risk of heart disease.

Fats known as '*trans*' fats

'*Trans*' fats are produced industrially by modifying the natural structure of a fatty acid. The *trans* fatty acids can be found in some margarines and spreads. There is some inconclusive evidence linking *trans* fatty acids with increased risk of atherosclerosis and some cancers; manufacturers are now producing margarines and spreads containing smaller amounts of *trans* fatty acids.

How do you use fats?

Fats are insoluble in water. Therefore, they have to be emulsified by bile salts to make them accessible to digestive enzymes. This occurs to a limited extent in your stomach, but is completed in your small intestine. The presence of undigested fat in your stomach delays the rate of emptying.

Fat is broken down by the enzymes into smaller compounds such as fatty acids and glycerols. These compounds form small particles called micelles, which are small enough to be absorbed through your gut wall. In your intestinal wall, the micelles are reassembled into larger compounds which are transported to your liver.

Your liver then produces lipoproteins, such as high-density lipoprotein (HDL), very-low-density lipoprotein (VLDL) and low-density lipoprotein (LDL). The amount and type of fat in your diet influence the ratio in which these lipoproteins are produced.

Absorption of fats into the body

The process of digestion of fats begins in the stomach and is completed in the small intestine. The constituent components of fat are transported to the liver where they are converted into lipoproteins, and thereafter stored or transported around the body.

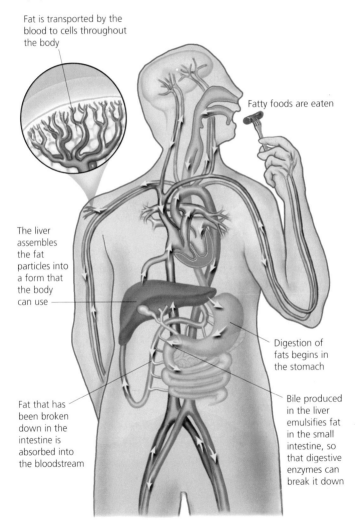

Fat is transported by the blood to cells throughout the body

Fatty foods are eaten

The liver assembles the fat particles into a form that the body can use

Digestion of fats begins in the stomach

Fat that has been broken down in the intestine is absorbed into the bloodstream

Bile produced in the liver emulsifies fat in the small intestine, so that digestive enzymes can break it down

How much do you need?

The Government guidelines on a balanced diet say that no more than 30 per cent of your total energy intake should come from fat. Saturated fat should not be responsible for more than 10 per cent of your total energy intake.

The recommended dietary intake of EFAs for adults is one to two per cent of the total energy intake and one per cent for children and babies. For adults this means two to five grams per day. However, the average daily intake for adults is actually 8 to 15 grams of EFAs per day. EFA deficiency is extremely rare in healthy individuals, but can occur in children and in patients requiring intravenous feeding.

Cholesterol

Cholesterol is used by your body to make steroid hormones and bile salts and to maintain the structure of cell membranes. However, raised blood cholesterol levels are associated with an increased risk of coronary heart disease (CHD). This is because cholesterol can be deposited in arteries, making them narrower – a condition known as atherosclerosis.

One or more blood vessels can become totally blocked, preventing blood from reaching the tissues served by the vessel. If the blood supply is stopped, the tissue dies. If the blocked vessel is one of the coronary arteries supplying blood to the heart, the result is a heart attack. Your likelihood of developing atherosclerosis is linked to several factors, including the amount of fat in your diet.

Atherosclerosis

Cholesterol is deposited on the inside of blood vessels, making them narrower and restricting blood flow.

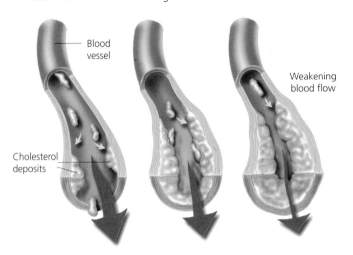

Blood vessel

Weakening blood flow

Cholesterol deposits

Diet and cholesterol levels

Although some foods are rich in cholesterol, most cholesterol (95 per cent) is made in your body. Your body makes cholesterol from saturated fat. The more saturated fat in your diet, the higher your blood cholesterol levels.

Polyunsaturated fats help to lower blood cholesterol. They trigger your liver to produce HDL, which reduces your risk of heart disease. Eating more high-fibre food, especially soluble fibre, also helps to reduce your cholesterol levels. Soluble fibre binds with cholesterol in bile, preventing its reabsorption by your body and increasing its excretion.

There has been a lot of interest in the so-called 'Mediterranean diet' eaten in southern Europe and north Africa, because people there have a lower rate

Heart disease risk factors

Several factors have been found to influence an individual's risk of developing heart disease. Some risks are unavoidable, others are not.

Avoidable

- Diet
- Smoking
- Obesity
- Stress
- Lack of exercise

Unavoidable

- Genetic disposition
- Gender
- Age
- High blood pressure

of coronary heart disease than people in the UK. This diet is high in monounsaturated fats. Studies suggest that these fats have little influence on blood cholesterol. The benefits of the 'Mediterranean diet' appear to derive from the fact that it is low in total fat and saturated fat and high in fruit, vegetables and wine.

Low levels of cholesterol have been linked to an increased risk of cancer. In fact, cancer rates are no higher in populations with low cholesterol levels than they are in those with high levels. Any disadvantages of a low cholesterol diet are outweighed by its benefits in reducing the risk of coronary heart disease.

Case study: risk of CHD

George, aged 50, moved home because of his job. The local health centre where he registered as a new patient required him to have a health check. This showed that he had several risk factors for coronary heart disease (CHD), including:

- a family history of CHD
- his age and gender
- his stressful job and lifestyle
- smoking
- being overweight
- raised blood pressure
- raised blood lipid levels.

The dietitian at the health centre suggested ways in which George could modify his lifestyle and reduce his risk factors for CHD. The first priority was to reduce George's weight, which he did by following a low-fat, high-fibre diet of no more than 1,500 kcal a day. This diet was designed to help him maintain a healthier weight and reduce his blood lipids. The practice nurse also encouraged George to take suitable exercise and advised him on how to cut his stress levels and stop smoking.

Six months later, George had reduced his weight by two stone and, as a result, his blood pressure was now normal. The changes in his diet and lifestyle resulted in a reduction in his blood lipids. The changes George had made over the previous six months had greatly reduced his risk factors for CHD and he was feeling fitter and more energetic than he had for a long time.

KEY POINTS

- Fat is an essential part of your diet

- Cutting down on your total fat intake, especially of saturated fat, is better than trying to substitute one kind of fat for another

- Fat should provide a maximum of 30 per cent of your total daily calories

Carbohydrates

Sugars, starches and fibre

Carbohydrates are your main source of energy. When carbohydrates are combined with oxygen (oxidised) in cells, carbon dioxide and water are formed and energy is released.

Glucose + Oxygen = Energy + Carbon dioxide + Water

Nutritionists classify carbohydrates into sugars, starches and fibre. The basic chemical structure of carbohydrates is a compound called a saccharide. Sugars are formed either from a single type, called a monosaccharide, or from two saccharides joined

Examples of the two types of sugars

Monosaccharides	Disaccharides
Glucose	Sucrose
Fructose	Lactose
Galactose	Maltose
Mannose	
Pentose	
Ribose	

together, forming a disaccharide. Many saccharides joined together make a polysaccharides. Starch is a polysaccharide.

How your body uses sugars

Sugars are important sources of dietary energy. Glucose is used as fuel by your body's cells, and your brain is almost entirely dependent on it for all its functions, including thinking.

Disaccharides are broken down by digestive enzymes in your intestine and absorbed as monosaccharides. For example, sucrose is broken down into glucose and fructose.

Excess sugars are stored in your liver as glycogen. These stores are mobilised if you're not getting enough energy from your diet or if energy is needed quickly for exercise. If the stores are full, sugars are converted into fat and stored in adipose tissue.

Your body is able to regulate the levels of glucose in your blood. If you eat a lot of carbohydrate, your pancreas produces more of the hormone insulin, which encourages the conversion of sugars into glycogen. This returns your blood glucose levels to normal. When you exercise, you use more glucose and need less insulin.

Where is sugar found?

Sugars are found in a variety of foods. Those occurring naturally in the structure of foods are called intrinsic sugars. Those added in the production process are called extrinsic sugars.

Glucose is found in small amounts in fruit and vegetables, such as grapes and onions, and, with fructose, it is one of the main constituents of honey. Free glucose is not a common natural sugar, but is

How the body uses carbohydrates

Carbohydrates are the body's main source of energy.

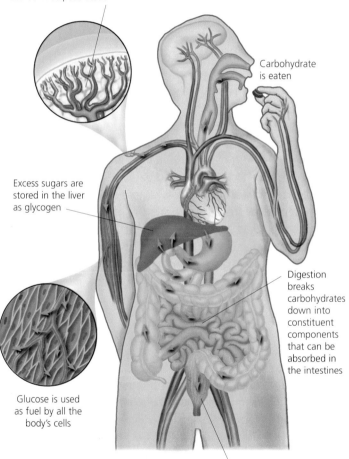

When no more sugars can be stored in the liver, they are converted into fat and stored in adipose tissue

Carbohydrate is eaten

Excess sugars are stored in the liver as glycogen

Digestion breaks carbohydrates down into constituent components that can be absorbed in the intestines

Glucose is used as fuel by all the body's cells

Undigested material is excreted

produced commercially from starch. Fructose is found in fruit, vegetables and honey. Galactose, combined with glucose, is found in milk.

Sucrose is the most commonly used disaccharide, and is extracted commercially from sugar beet or sugar cane. It is present in fruit and vegetables, but table sugar, which is 99 per cent pure sucrose, is the major source in the diet.

Maltose is produced commercially by breaking down starch. It is present in malted wheat and barley, which are used to produce malted foods and in the brewing industry to make beer. Lactose is found naturally only in milk and milk products. It consists of glucose and galactose.

Food manufacturers use many sugars in foods. All of the following are sugars or sugar-related products: glucose, fructose, galactose, lactose, invert sugar, mannose, pentose, ribose, sucrose, maltose, sorbitol, mannitol, dulcitol, inositol, corn syrup, trehalose, raffinose, stachyose, vernanose and fructans.

Commercial sugar comes in many forms, including white, granulated, caster, icing, demerara, cane, soft brown, dark brown, treacle, golden syrup, molasses and cubes. The stage and type of processing determine the colour and form of the sugar. None of these sugars contains substantial amounts of any other nutrients.

Sugar alcohols, such as sorbitol, are compounds that are sweet but have the same chemical structure as alcohol. Sorbitol is found naturally in some fruits, such as cherries, but it is also made commercially from glucose.

How much sugar do you need?
Recent surveys show that sugars provide 18 per cent of the total energy intake of the average adult. The intake

of 'refined' or 'added' sugars may contribute to the development of obesity and may limit the intake of other more beneficial foods, especially fibre. Sugars contribute energy but no other nutrients to the diet, and are therefore often called 'empty calories'. Current thinking is that we should reduce the amount of energy from sugar to no more than 10 per cent of our energy intake.

Sugars and dental disease

Sugars in the diet have been linked to dental disease. Dental plaque is the white layer that builds up on teeth between brushings. Plaque is made of bacteria, water, polysaccharides and sometimes dead cells from your mouth. It collects in areas that are difficult to clean, which are often called food traps. Sugars from food pass into the plaque and are changed into acid by bacteria. The acid starts to dissolve the hard enamel coating of your teeth, causing tooth decay or dental caries. When the acid is neutralised, your tooth can heal, but a frequent intake of sugars maintains the acid environment, stopping the healing process.

People who eat large amounts of refined sugars, such as sucrose, have the most dental decay. The more frequent the intake of refined sugars, the greater the number of cavities found.

There is no evidence to suggest that intrinsic sugars, such as fructose in fruit and lactose in milk and milk products, have any adverse effects on teeth. However, the use of fruit juices in comforters (dummies), which maintain prolonged periods of contact with teeth, can contribute to decay. There is strong evidence to suggest that extrinsic sugars, such as sucrose, are involved in the development of dental decay.

Tooth decay

Bacteria on the teeth and gums convert the sugar in the mouth
to acid, which erodes the hard enamel covering the tooth and
invades the softer dentin.

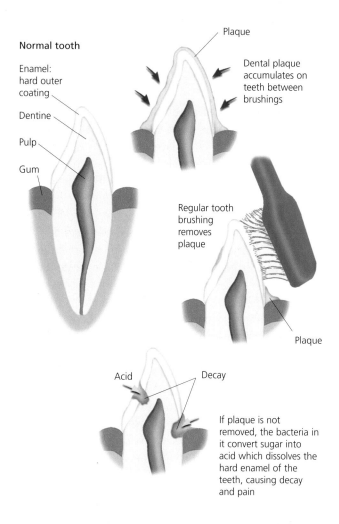

Normal tooth

Enamel:
hard outer
coating

Dentine

Pulp

Gum

Plaque

Dental plaque
accumulates on
teeth between
brushings

Regular tooth
brushing
removes
plaque

Plaque

Acid   Decay

If plaque is not
removed, the bacteria in
it convert sugar into
acid which dissolves the
hard enamel of the
teeth, causing decay
and pain

Starches

Starchy foods are an important part of your diet. In some parts of the world, starch provides up to 80 per cent of the total energy intake. In the UK, starch provides about 24 per cent of the total energy intake.

What is starch?

Starch is a large, complex compound (a polysaccharide) made up of many glucose molecules. The glucose can combine in many different ways or patterns, and this affects the rate at which you digest and absorb starch. The more complicated the pattern, the more resistant the starch will be to digestion.

Raw starch is very difficult to digest. Processing, such as cooking, can change the patterns of glucose molecules, making the starch more digestible. Heating starch in water causes it to swell and thicken, and then the digestive enzyme amylase can break it down into glucose, which can be absorbed into your body.

Where does starch come from?

In the UK, the major sources of starches in the diet are staple foods such as potatoes, cereal grains (wheat, barley, maize, oats and rye) and rice. The following ingredients are also forms of starch: amylopectin, dextrins, maltodextrins and glycogen.

How much do you need?

There is no official recommendation for starches, but a healthy diet should provide an average of 37 per cent of energy from starches, intrinsic sugars (which occur naturally in produce) and milk sugars. The same is true for children over two years. The best nourishment for babies is breast milk, which does not contain starch.

Diabetes

Rapidly absorbed carbohydrates, such as sucrose, result in high glucose levels in the blood. Healthy people are able to cope with this by adjusting their insulin production accordingly. Insulin is a hormone, secreted by the pancreas, that helps to move glucose from the blood into the body's cells.

If you have diabetes, this mechanism doesn't work. The aim of diabetic control is to maintain blood glucose levels within normal limits. People with diabetes either do not produce insulin and need to inject it (type 1 or insulin-dependent diabetes mellitus) or produce insulin but are resistant to its action (type 2 or non-insulin-dependent diabetes mellitus). Either way, they can't deal effectively with a rapid rise in blood glucose. High levels of glucose in the blood result in the acute symptoms of diabetes, such as thirst and increased urination and, in the long term, in complications such as eye, nerve and circulatory disorders.

Not all carbohydrates are potentially harmful to people with diabetes. For example, starches are important to people with diabetes because they do not cause rapid changes in blood glucose levels, yet provide energy and fibre.

Foods containing a high proportion of starch

- Potatoes
- Pasta
- Rice
- Popcorn
- Bread
- Baked beans
- Biscuits

Sorbitol is often used in products manufactured for people with diabetes. It is 60 per cent as sweet as sucrose, is absorbed slowly from the gut and is then stored as fructose in the liver. It has less effect on blood glucose levels than sucrose. However, sorbitol has more calories per gram and too much of it can give you diarrhoea. People with diabetes don't actually need a sucrose substitute and they could also do without the extra calories that it provides. Diabetes UK does not recommend the use of special diabetic food products to its members.

Fibre or non-starch polysaccharides

Fibre was originally called roughage and is now referred to as non-starch polysaccharides (NSPs). Technically, dietary fibre is difficult to define and analysing foods for their fibre content can be problematic. Government bodies have recommended that the term 'non-starch polysaccharides' be used in food labelling. However, as fibre is the term that most people know, it is used throughout this book.

What is fibre and what does it do?

Fibre is the major component of plant cell walls and is resistant to enzymes that digest food. Most of the fibre in the diet comes from fruit, vegetables and cereals. In wheat, maize and rice, the fibre is mainly insoluble, whereas, in oats, barley and rye, it is mainly soluble. In fruit and vegetables, the ratio of insoluble to soluble fibre is variable. Each kind of fibre plays a different role in digestion.

Insoluble fibre increases the bulk and wetness of faeces. It therefore prevents and relieves constipation by holding water in your bowel. The increased bulk speeds up the transit time of faeces and reduces the pressure in your bowel. The reduction in pressure helps

Soluble and insoluble fibre sources

Insoluble fibre passes through the intestine unchanged whereas soluble fibre is partly broken down by bacteria in the intestine. The following foods are examples of each type:

Soluble fibre
- Beans, for example, baked beans
- Lentils
- Peas
- Oats
- Oranges
- Apples

Insoluble fibre
- Wholemeal bread
- Wholemeal breakfast cereals
- Wholemeal biscuits and crisp breads
- Brown rice
- Wheat bran
- Oats

prevent a condition called diverticular disease (for more details, see pages 12–13).

Soluble fibre has little effect on stool bulk. However, it binds bile acids, which are rich in cholesterol. The cholesterol found in bile is usually reabsorbed into your body. Soluble fibre prevents this reabsorption, so more cholesterol is lost in the faeces and less is taken back into your bloodstream. This can be important in the prevention of coronary heart disease.

The digestion and absorption of carbohydrates are slower if there is a good supply of fibre in your diet.

This results in a more gradual release of glucose into your blood, which is especially important for people with diabetes. Fibre makes you feel full because, once it has absorbed water, it has a larger bulk.

How much fibre do you need?

A recent Government panel recommended that the adult diet should contain 12 to 24 grams of fibre per day from a variety of sources. This amount could be provided by five portions of fruit and vegetables per day.

There is no specific recommendation for children besides suggesting that fibre intake should be related to body size, so children need proportionately less than adults. Children under the age of two should not be given fibre at the expense of energy-rich foods that are needed for growth.

Generally, foods rich in fibre have more bulk, are less energy dense and are more likely to reduce hunger than fibre-free foods. This suggests that they can play a useful role in weight-reducing diets.

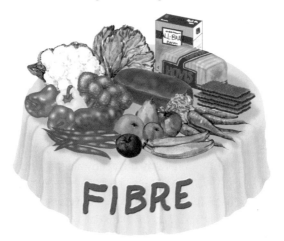

Fruit, vegetables and cereals are the main sources of fibre.

Glycaemic index

The glycaemic index (GI) is a way of ranking foods, depending on the type of carbohydrate that they contain and the effect that they have on blood sugar levels. Low GI foods are slowly absorbed. Quickly absorbed foods have a high GI.

Low GI foods can help even out blood glucose levels in people with diabetes and may help people on a weight-reducing diet. Diets with high GI may increase the risk of heart disease.

The way in which foods are manufactured and cooked will affect their GI. Try to have a combination of carbohydrates in a meal so that your diet has a low-to-medium GI.

How the glycaemic index (GI) works

The glycaemic index (GI) runs from 0 to 100 and usually uses glucose – which has a GI value of 100 – as the reference. The effect that other foods have on blood sugar levels is then compared with this. In simple terms, the GI tells us whether a food raises blood sugar levels dramatically (high GI value), moderately (medium GI value) or a little bit (low GI level).

Low GI	Medium GI	High GI
Red kidney beans	Porridge	Raisins
Wholemeal spaghetti	Digestive biscuits	Chocolate biscuits
Milk	Crisps	Honey
Apples	Carrots	White rice
Soya beans	Grapes	Cornflakes

Glycaemic load

The glycaemic load of a food considers the combined effect of the amount of a food and its glycaemic index on blood sugar levels. A healthy diet should have a low glycaemic load.

Case study: type 2 diabetes

Mary was a keen tennis player until she retired. She then became more sedentary and gradually put on weight. She noticed that she was always tired and thought that it was, at least partly, because she had to go to the toilet at least twice during the night. Eventually, Mary consulted her GP, who asked her for a urine sample. Using a simple dipstick test, the doctor found that Mary had a lot of glucose in her urine. He then did a finger-prick test, which showed that her blood glucose level was also high.

Mary was diagnosed with type 2 diabetes. This could be treated by a change of diet, with or without tablets. A dietitian analysed Mary's normal diet and felt that Mary was eating too much refined sugar and fat. She suggested a healthy eating plan. Mary needed to control her energy intake so as to lose weight. She needed to eat a variety of foods and have regular meals and snacks. She needed to eat less fat, eat more fruit and vegetables – ideally five portions a day – and include more fibre in her diet.

The dietitian also told Mary that there was no need to use products made especially for people with diabetes. These contain ingredients that are low in glucose but high in other refined carbohydrates, or they contain sweeteners such as sorbitol.

Once Mary's weight returned to normal, her diabetes improved greatly. She was able to monitor her glucose levels by using simple blood and urine tests. When Mary was feeling less tired, she joined the local tennis club. Regular exercise improved her general health and made it easier for her to control her blood glucose levels.

KEY POINTS

- Carbohydrate is an important source of energy in your diet

- Try to eat more carbohydrate foods and reduce the fat content of your diet

- Complex carbohydrates (starches and fibre) make you feel full

Vitamins
and minerals

Micronutrients

Vitamins and minerals are an essential part of a balanced diet. They are needed by your body in minute amounts for many vital chemical reactions, such as extracting energy from food. They are often called micronutrients. A lack of vitamins or minerals can lead to ill-health and cause deficiency diseases.

Vitamins

Vitamins were originally known by letters of the alphabet, but now researchers and other health professionals more often use their chemical names. Since the end of the nineteenth century, the understanding of vitamins and their role in human health and deficiency syndromes has increased greatly. Recent research has extended this knowledge to show that vitamins may also play a part in preventing diseases such as cancer.

What are vitamins?

Vitamins are complex chemical substances. Most can't be made in your body, so you have to obtain them from food. One exception is vitamin D, which can be made in your skin on exposure to sunlight. Bacteria, which aren't part of your body but live inside your gut, can also make some vitamins.

Vitamins can be split into two groups: water soluble and fat soluble. Water-soluble vitamins can be dissolved in water and, therefore, are found in non-fatty, water-rich foods such as fruit and vegetables. Fat-soluble vitamins are found in fatty foods, as their chemical structures allow them to be dissolved in fat.

Some vitamins, particularly water-soluble vitamins, are gradually lost from foods over time. For this reason, the fresher the foods, and the less they are cooked, the better the supplies of vitamins available. Vitamin C, for example, is destroyed by heat, and vitamin B$_1$ (thiamine) is sensitive to light. Frozen vegetables are often better sources of vitamins because they are frozen very soon after harvest and the vitamins are preserved. Fresh vegetables may be in transit or in the shop for days before being sold and then may be stored for some time at home before they are used.

Water-soluble vitamins

Common name	Chemical name
Vitamin C	Ascorbic acid
Vitamin B$_1$	Thiamine
Vitamin B$_2$	Riboflavin
Vitamin B$_6$	Pyridoxine, pyridoxal, pyridoxamine
Vitamin B$_{12}$	Cyanocobalamin, cobalamin
Folate	Folic acid
Niacin	Nicotinic acid, nicotinamide, niacinamide
Pantothenic acid	
Biotin	

How much do you need?

Only small amounts of each vitamin are required each day. There are recommended daily allowances (RDAs) for several vitamins in the UK, including thiamine, folate, riboflavin, niacin, vitamins A, B_6, B_{12}, C and D. The RDA is the required level of intake needed to maintain good health. It varies between different groups of people; infants, children, elderly people, adults and pregnant and breast-feeding women all require different amounts. For more details on vitamin supplements, see 'Dietary supplements, alternative diets and "health foods"' on page 116.

Water-soluble vitamins

Vitamin C (ascorbic acid)

Vitamin C helps to maintain your skin and connective tissue and helps iron to be absorbed from your gut. People who don't get enough vitamin C develop a condition called scurvy, which causes fatigue, bleeding and poor wound healing. Vitamin C deficiency is rare in healthy individuals, but can affect people with illnesses such as cancer, malabsorption syndromes and alcoholism, or those who are being fed intravenously.

Vitamin C is found in fruit and vegetables, especially citrus fruit, tomatoes, spinach, potatoes and broccoli. It is easily destroyed by heat and light, so foods rich in vitamin C should be stored in a cool, dark place, and prepared and cooked as quickly as possible.

Taking high doses of vitamin C (several times more than the RDA) has been claimed to reduce your chances of catching the common cold. Apart from its now accepted role in preventing damage caused by free radicals (see page 71), other claims for vitamin C have not been proved. Taking too much can be harmful, causing diarrhoea and kidney stones. As vitamin C increases iron uptake, taking too much can also lead to iron overload.

Vitamin B$_1$ (thiamine)

Thiamine helps to break down carbohydrate, fat and alcohol. People who have a thiamine deficiency (known as beri-beri) cannot process carbohydrates or fat properly and develop a range of symptoms including cardiac and neurological problems. In the UK, the condition mainly affects people with chronic disease, malabsorption problems or anorexia. Chronic binge-drinking alcoholics can also develop thiamine deficiency.

Most of the thiamine in the diet comes from fortified cereals and bread. Other major sources are offal, pork, nuts and legumes (peas and beans).

Large doses of thiamine, in excess of three grams per day, may cause headaches, insomnia, weakness and skin problems.

Vitamin B$_2$ (riboflavin)

Your body needs vitamin B$_2$ to extract energy from fat, protein and carbohydrate in food. The main sources of riboflavin are dairy products, meat, fish, asparagus, broccoli, poultry and spinach. Some cereals are fortified with riboflavin. Riboflavin is sensitive to ultraviolet light.

Riboflavin deficiency can cause skin disorders, especially in and around the mouth. There is no evidence that riboflavin has toxic effects on the body, or that large doses do any good.

Vitamin B$_6$ (pyridoxine)

Pyridoxine is essential for the metabolism of proteins and haemoglobin (the oxygen-carrying red pigment in your blood), and so the quantity that you need depends on how much protein you eat. Pyridoxine deficiency causes skin problems in and around the mouth and neurological problems, but this rarely affects healthy people.

Bacteria in your gut make pyridoxine, some of which is absorbed through your intestinal wall. Poultry, fish, pork, eggs and offal are rich sources of pyridoxine, as are oats, peanuts and soybeans.

Pyridoxine supplements are taken by many women to treat premenstrual symptoms, but there is no conclusive evidence showing that they have a beneficial effect.

Vitamin B_{12} (cyanocobalamin)
Cyanocobalamin is involved in the production of red blood cells. Foods derived from animals (including dairy products) are a good source of vitamin B_{12}. Strict vegetarians and vegans may need to take supplements to make up for any deficiency in their diets.

To be able to use vitamin B_{12}, your stomach must produce a substance called intrinsic factor. People who have a stomach disorder preventing them from making enough intrinsic factor cannot absorb vitamin B_{12} properly; they develop pernicious anaemia.

There is no evidence that taking large doses of vitamin B_{12} does any harm.

Folate
Folate (folic acid) is essential for the normal formation of red blood cells. People with folic acid deficiency may develop a condition called megaloblastic anaemia in which the red blood cells are enlarged. Sources of folates include liver, yeast extract and green, leafy vegetables.

A good supply is particularly important for women who are planning to conceive and those who are in the first three months of pregnancy, when the recommended intake is 400 micrograms per day. Folate has been shown to reduce the risk of having a baby with a neural tube defect such as spina bifida.

High intakes of folate are not dangerous, but they may affect the absorption of zinc and interfere with tests used to diagnose vitamin B_{12} deficiency. Unless you are planning to conceive or are in early pregnancy, there are no proven benefits from taking large doses.

Niacin

Niacin is involved in fat metabolism and is necessary to maintain the condition of your skin. Niacin deficiency is rare in developed countries, but in Asia and Africa it results in a condition called pellagra, which can be fatal if untreated.

Meat is a good source of niacin and cereals provide moderate amounts. Niacin can also be made in your body from the amino acid tryptophan. Excess niacin is excreted in your urine, although very large doses can cause liver problems.

Pantothenic acid and biotin

Pantothenic acid and biotin are involved in fat and carbohydrate metabolism and are found in foods derived from animal sources (including dairy products) and in cereals and pulses. There are no recommended intakes and they are not known to be toxic.

Fat-soluble vitamins

Vitamin A (retinol)

Vitamin A can be made in your body from substances called beta-carotenes, which are found in dark-green, orange and yellow vegetables such as spinach and carrots. Retinol is obtained from animal sources, such as meat and dairy products, and is added to margarine in the UK. Deficiency is rare in the UK, but is a major cause of blindness in children in some developing countries.

Retinol is toxic in large doses (300 milligrams in adults and 100 milligrams in children) but most damage is done by accumulation. Toxicity can lead to liver and bone damage and cause birth defects. You shouldn't take supplements or eat large quantities of liver just before or during pregnancy.

Vitamin D (calciferol)

Vitamin D is important in the growth and maintenance of bone because it controls the absorption of calcium and phosphorus, which are essential in bone metabolism. Children who don't get enough vitamin D develop rickets; adults develop weak, soft bones, a condition known as osteomalacia.

Fat-soluble vitamins

Common name	Chemical name
Vitamin A	Retinol, retinoic acid, beta-carotene (the latter is converted to vitamin A in the body)
Vitamin D	Calciferols
Vitamin E	Tocopherols
Vitamin K	Phylloquinone, menaquinone, menadione

Sources of vitamin D include fatty fish, such as pilchards, sardines, mackerel and tuna, eggs and fortified foods such as margarine and some breakfast cereals. Vitamin D can be made in your skin by ultraviolet rays in sunlight.

Deficiency is rare in the UK, but does occur in people who have little vitamin D in their diet and whose skins are rarely exposed to sunlight – for example, elderly people and some Asian women. Large doses can lead to high blood levels of calcium, especially in children, and may result in bone malformations, although this is extremely rare. There are no dietary recommendations for adults who have a normal lifestyle involving exposure to sunlight.

Vitamin E (tocopherol)

Tocopherol acts as an antioxidant, which means that it stops your body's cells being attacked by chemicals called oxygen-generated free radicals. Vitamin E is important in maintaining the structure of lipids (fats) in your body and any structures, such as membranes surrounding cells, that are rich in lipids. Deficiency in humans is rare, occurring only in premature babies and in people with some malabsorption syndromes. Dietary sources include vegetable oils, nuts, vegetables and cereals. There is little evidence of tocopherol toxicity.

Vitamin K (phylloquinone, menaquinone and menadione)

The three forms of vitamin K are slightly different in their chemical make-up. Vitamin K is involved in blood clotting and a deficiency will lead to bruising and excessive bleeding. Deficiency is rare except in newborn babies and people who have diseases affecting vitamin absorption or metabolism. Dark-green, leafy vegetables are the major sources in the diet, although bacteria in your gut can make vitamin K, which is absorbed into your blood.

Minerals

Minerals are single chemical elements that are involved in various processes in your body. If you eat a varied diet, you should obtain all the minerals that you need. Unlike vitamins, minerals do not deteriorate during storage or cooking, so mineral deficiency is rare, except in people being fed intravenously or who have certain diseases. One exception is iron deficiency, which is often the result of blood loss or may develop in people who are strict vegetarians or vegans.

Your body is able to adapt to make the most of its mineral supplies; for example, your iron absorption increases if your diet is poor in iron. This is why taking mineral supplements may cause problems: overloading with one mineral may decrease the absorption of another that is absorbed in your body via the same route.

Sodium, potassium and chromium

Sodium, potassium and chromium are also referred to, in solution, as electrolytes. They are widely distributed throughout your body and have many functions, including maintaining your nerves in proper working order. Deficiencies and high levels of these chemicals are usually caused by a problem with a person's metabolism – for example, certain diseases or dehydration caused by excessive vomiting. Electrolytes are readily available in animal and vegetable foods.

Other minerals and trace elements

Other minerals and trace elements used by your body include aluminium, antimony, boron, bromine, cadmium, lithium, nickel, sulphur and strontium. They are readily available in your diet and, as their name suggests, are only necessary in trace (tiny) quantities.

Antioxidants and disease prevention

Recently, there has been evidence that some vitamins and the mineral selenium may act as defences against certain diseases. When oxygen is used in chemical reactions in your body, it produces, as a byproduct, potentially harmful chemicals called free radicals. These cause tissue damage and may lead to some conditions such as heart disease and some cancers. Your body has

Antioxidants and free radicals

Free radicals are potentially harmful chemicals that are produced as a byproduct of metabolism. Antioxidants are thought to be able to inhibit the action of free radicals.

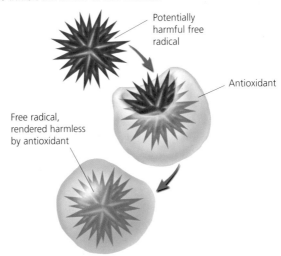

Potentially harmful free radical

Antioxidant

Free radical, rendered harmless by antioxidant

Sources of antioxidants

Antioxidant	Present in
Vitamin A	Dairy products, oily fish (herring, sardines, tuna) and fish oils
Beta-carotene	Fruit and vegetables
Vitamin C	Fruit and vegetables (spinach, tomato, potato, broccoli, strawberry, orange and citrus)
Vitamin E	Fruit, vegetables, cereals, dairy, nuts, eggs
Selenium	Cereal grains, meat, fish
Lycopene	Cooked/processed tomatoes from sauces

powerful defence mechanisms to prevent such damage, but in some cases (for example, in smokers), this mechanism is impaired.

Antioxidants, such as vitamin A, beta-carotene, vitamins C and E, selenium and lycopene, are able to stop the action of free radicals. Dietary sources of antioxidants are fruit and vegetables, nuts, cereals and fish (and their oils).

Diseases linked to free radical damage occur for many reasons. However, eating a diet that is rich in antioxidant foods can reduce your risk of developing them. A recent Government committee has recommended that the best way of ensuring that you get enough of the relevant nutrients is to eat five portions of fruit and vegetables a day.

Some reports have suggested that people who eat large quantities of red meat are particularly at risk, although the reason for this is unclear; it may be that people who eat a lot of meat also tend to eat smaller quantities of fruit and vegetables and are not protected against free radical damage.

Case study: osteomalacia

Henry (aged 80) lived alone and was totally housebound. A helper shopped and cleaned for him and prepared a snack lunch each day. Henry rarely cooked a meal and found fruit difficult to eat because of his dentures. He dismissed the aches and pains in his bones and muscles as 'old age'.

One morning, Henry slipped getting out of bed. His home help found him on the floor, unable to move. At the hospital, it was discovered that he'd fractured the top of his thigh bone, a type of fracture that is most common in elderly people. Blood tests showed that Henry had abnormally low levels of calcium and vitamin D. A bone scan confirmed that Henry was suffering from osteomalacia. Undoubtedly, his poor diet contributed to his condition, but an important factor was his lack of exposure to sunlight, which triggers the production of vitamin D.

A dietitian gave Henry advice on which foods to eat. Social services arranged transport to a local day care centre, where he would have a nourishing meal. Going out regularly would increase Henry's exposure to sunlight, improving his bone condition.

KEY POINTS

■ A balanced diet provides all the necessary vitamins and minerals for healthy adults

■ The benefits of large doses of vitamins (much higher than the recommended daily allowance) are not proven; large doses of fat-soluble vitamins can actually be harmful

■ Some people are at risk of a vitamin or mineral deficiency (for example, pregnant women and vegetarians), and may benefit from supplements of the correct dosage

■ Research has found links between a low vitamin and mineral intake and heart disease and some cancers; it is believed that five portions of fruit and vegetables per day can reduce the risk of developing these diseases

■ Taking folate supplements (400 micrograms per day) in pregnancy reduces the risk of having a baby with spina bifida

Healthy eating

A balanced approach

The key to eating a healthy diet is to have a balanced approach to food. There is no such thing as a 'good' or 'bad' food. It is important to view your diet as a whole. Only if your diet is unbalanced and contains too much of a 'less good' food will it become unhealthy.

No food has to be forbidden in a healthy diet, except on medical grounds, although some are best kept as an occasional treat. If you deny yourself a particular favourite food, you are more likely to become obsessed with it and crave it all the time. When you do succumb, you're more likely to over-indulge than if you include it in your diet every now and again.

The five food groups

There are five food groups:

1 Fruit and vegetables

2 Bread, cereals, pasta and potatoes (carbohydrates)

3 Meat, fish and alternatives (protein foods)

4 Milk and dairy foods

5 Foods containing fat or sugar.

To achieve a balanced diet, you should choose a variety of foods from the first four groups. This will supply you with enough of the various nutrients that your body needs. Foods in the fifth group do not always provide a wide variety of nutrients, but can make your diet more enjoyable. They should be eaten only in moderation. Don't worry if you can't get this balance right with every meal, but aim to do so over the course of a few days.

Aim to have three meals a day with small snacks in between if you want them. Snacks don't have to be high in calories or fat – fruit or a couple of wholemeal biscuits is a better bet. Breakfast is an important meal and shouldn't be missed. The longer you go between meals or snacks, the more likely you are to overeat when you next get the chance.

Foods should be included in your diet in relative proportions. You don't need to measure quantities of

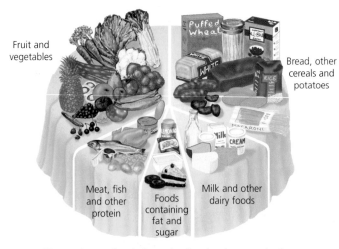

Fruit and vegetables

Bread, other cereals and potatoes

Meat, fish and other protein

Foods containing fat and sugar

Milk and other dairy foods

Aim to choose foods from the five food groups in the approximate proportions shown here.

Healthy snacks

Snacks can be healthy and nutritious as well as easy to prepare. Include foods that are low in sugar, fat and salt, and high in fibre. The most healthy snack and easiest to prepare is fresh fruit.

- Fresh fruit
- Dried fruit (be careful if watching calories)
- Raw chopped vegetables, for example, carrot or celery sticks
- Plain popcorn
- Plain scone or currant bun
- Low-fat yoghurt or fromage frais
- Bread sticks

different foods accurately, except on medical advice, when your eating pattern should be supervised by a qualified dietitian or a doctor.

Your eating plan
Fruit and vegetables

Fruit and vegetables provide vitamins, minerals and fibre. The fibre can reduce constipation and help to prevent bowel disease and coronary heart disease. Fruit and vegetables are good sources of the antioxidants vitamins A and C. Recent research has shown that these substances may help prevent other diseases including some cancers. Frozen, dried and tinned fruit and vegetables are just as nutritious as fresh foods. Adults should aim to have five portions of fruit and vegetables every day. Children can be given smaller portions according to their appetite.

What is a portion?

Nutrition professionals often advise the inclusion of a certain number of portions of fruit and vegetables in the diet. This chart shows examples of the portion sizes of particular foods.

Food	Portion
Apple, banana, orange	1 fruit
Plums	2 fruits
Dried fruit	1 tablespoon
Grapes, cherries	1 cupful
Fruit juice	1 small glass
Vegetables	2 tablespoons
Salad	1 dessert bowlful

Carbohydrates

It is important to eat plenty of carbohydrates, as they are good sources of energy, fibre, calcium, iron and B vitamins. Wholemeal bread and pasta and brown rice are particularly good sources of fibre. As well as preventing constipation and bowel disease, eating lots of fibre will make you feel full, helping you to stop overeating. High-fibre diets can also lower blood cholesterol, reducing the risk of coronary heart disease.

Fat

Fat is an essential part of your diet but you don't need very much. It provides energy, essential fatty acids and vitamins, and makes food tastier to eat. However, high levels are associated with coronary heart disease and obesity, so it is important to cut down your intake, especially when it comes to saturated fat.

You can do this by eating less 'visible' fat – such as

fatty meats and eggs – and using less fat and oil for cooking and spreading. Food manufacturers offer a wide choice of low-fat products.

Some products, such as cakes or biscuits, contain 'invisible' fats, so you need to read food labels carefully. Try using products that are high in polyunsaturated fats and low in saturated fats.

Eating oily fish twice a week can help to prevent heart disease. Oily fish include salmon, kippers, tuna, sardines, pilchards, mackerel, herring, trout and anchovies.

Sugary food and drinks

These contain calories and no other nutrients, so try not to have too many of them. They are particularly harmful to your teeth and are best eaten at the end of meals.

Alcohol

Drinking one to two units of alcohol per day has been shown to be beneficial to health by reducing the risk of coronary heart disease. However, drinking large quantities of alcohol increases the risks to your health, and this applies even if you abstain all week and then binge at weekends.

Salt

Although we all need a little salt in our diet there is now evidence to suggest that sodium, found in salt, is associated with high blood pressure (also known as hypertension). Hypertension can increase the risk of heart disease and stroke. Try to reduce your salt intake by adding less salt to food when cooking and at the table, consuming fewer salted foods and choosing processed food with 'low salt' or 'reduced salt' options.

A healthy weight
The right weight for you

You can find the appropriate weight for your height by using the chart on page 81. People in the 'correct weight' band on the chart have a body mass index (BMI) of between 20 and 25. To calculate your BMI, divide your weight in kilograms by your height in metres squared.

If your BMI is less than 18.5, you are underweight. You should be careful not to lose any more weight and should consult your doctor. If your BMI is 18.5 to 25, your weight is in proportion to your height. If your BMI is 25 to 30, you are a bit overweight. Unless your health is affected (arthritis, for example, is made worse by excess weight), then you don't need to worry.

If your BMI is above 30, you are overweight and should consider losing weight – otherwise your health will suffer. At BMI values greater than 30, there is an increased risk of many diseases. These include coronary heart disease (CHD), high blood pressure (a risk factor for CHD), some cancers, diabetes mellitus, musculo-skeletal problems, reproductive disorders and gallbladder disease.

If you are concerned about your weight, your GP will be able to advise you and may refer you to a dietitian or the practice nurse.

Losing weight wisely

To lose weight you should eat a high-fibre, low-fat diet that follows the given guidelines but has smaller portions. Once you have reached a comfortable weight that gives you a BMI below 30, you should eat a balanced diet and not have too many calories.

Exercise is an important part of weight maintenance. It does not have to be strenuous but just enough to

What should you weigh?

- The body mass index (BMI) is a useful measure of healthy weight
- Find out your height in metres and weight in kilograms
- Calculate your BMI like this

$$BMI = \frac{\text{Your weight (kg)}}{[\text{Your height (metres)} \times \text{Your height (metres)}]}$$

e.g. $24.8 = \dfrac{70}{[1.68 \times 1.68]}$

- You are recommended to try to maintain a BMI in the range 20–25
- The chart below is an easier way of estimating your BMI. Read off your height and your weight. The point where the lines cross in the chart indicates your BMI

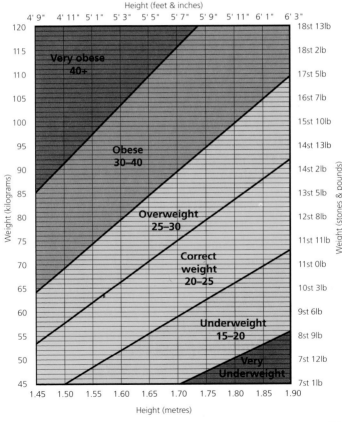

make you feel slightly out of breath – a brisk walk, for example. Aim to exercise for 20 to 30 minutes two or three times a week. Many GPs can now prescribe a fitness programme at the local sports centre. This may be available free or for a reduced fee.

The recommended rate of weight loss is one pound per week. If you lose weight too quickly, you may lose body tissues that are not associated with the excess weight (that is, fat-free mass). This will make it harder for you to maintain your new weight.

You'll lose more weight when you first start to diet because your body uses up its stores of glycogen from your liver and muscle. Glycogen is stored with water so, as you use glycogen, you excrete a large amount of water in your urine. Glycogen is usually used up by the end of the first or second week of your diet.

How much weight you lose in this initial stage will depend on the energy and carbohydrate content of your diet before you started. If you were eating a diet low in carbohydrates, your glycogen stores will be smaller than those of someone who eats large amounts.

The distribution of fat in the body is also important. People with relatively large waists (apple shaped) are more at risk of health problems than those with relatively large hips (pear shaped). A quick reference guide to the risk for your waist circumference can be obtained from Ashwell Associates (see 'Useful information', page 126).

Feeding children

Up to the age of four months, breast or formula milk provides all the nutrients that a baby needs. You can begin to introduce solids around this time, starting with baby rice and then puréed fruit and vegetables. Over the following weeks and months, you can gradually increase the amount and texture, so that, at 12 months, your child is eating a varied diet of three meals and two or three snacks a day. Gradually introducing different textures will encourage your child to chew.

Whether you opt for bought or home-made food is a matter of personal choice. Preparing baby and toddler meals doesn't have to be time-consuming and fiddly, and is certainly less expensive. For example, you can make extra of a particular dish, such as fruit and vegetables, when cooking for the rest of your family. The extra portions can be puréed and frozen. Remember, however, not to add salt or sugar until your child's portion has been put into a separate dish. Keep the portions small when you first start – ice cube trays make ideal containers for freezing foods. That way, not much is wasted if your baby doesn't like a particular food. An older toddler can be served with the rest of your family and his or her food simply mashed in the serving bowl.

Although children under two years should not eat too much fat, there is no need for them to be on a low-fat diet. They need a lot of energy to grow, some of which can be provided by fat. By the age of five, your child should be eating a balanced diet similar to that eaten by the rest of your family.

Fussy eaters

Some children won't eat a variety of foods or at times appear to eat very little. Although it is very frustrating and upsetting for you as a parent, the best approach is to stay as calm as you can and not give your child too much attention. If you allow eating to become an issue, you will simply make the problem worse. You may be able to avoid this situation if you give your child a wide variety of foods and try to make mealtimes a relaxing and enjoyable experience.

If you are concerned about your child's diet, a referral from your GP to a paediatric dietitian may be helpful. She will be able to assess your child's diet and, with the doctor, his or her growth and development. Most fussy children are actually growing well and require little or no intervention from health professionals. Try to be patient and keep reminding yourself that most children grow out of this phase.

Case study: obesity

Six months after the birth of her baby, Jane started to notice that she got breathless walking upstairs and was finding coping with him physically more difficult. At 5 feet 4 inches (1.6 metres) and 13 stone 7 pounds (86 kilograms), she was clearly overweight, so her health visitor suggested that Jane should talk to the practice nurse. The practice nurse calculated that Jane had a BMI of 33.6, meaning she was officially classified as obese. The normal weight range for a woman of Jane's height is 8 to 10 stones (51 to 64 kilograms). After talking to Jane about her lifestyle and eating patterns, the practice nurse was able to agree on some changes with her:

- Eat three meals a day plus small snacks if necessary

- Cut down on fatty foods, using low-fat foods if necessary

- Increase the amount of fibre in her diet

- Have at least five portions of fruit and vegetables each day

- Avoid fried food and cut out sugar as far as possible
- Aim for a total intake of 1,400 kcal a day.

The aim was for Jane to lose approximately one pound per week after the initial period of rapid weight loss. Once her weight had dropped, Jane should try to follow the same healthy eating guidelines to ensure that she didn't immediately put back what she'd lost. She lost four pounds in the first week of her diet and was surprised that she didn't feel she was depriving herself of any foods. She subsequently lost between one and one and a half pounds a week for the next month and soon felt confident to carry on without making the weekly visits to the practice nurse. She agreed to a check-up every three months to see that she is not regaining weight, but she is still heading for her target weight of about 10 stone (64 kg).

KEY POINTS

- Have three meals a day and don't skip breakfast

- There is no reason to avoid snacks

- Eat more fibre and carbohydrate and reduce fat

- Eat five portions of fruit and vegetables per day

- Food should be a pleasure, not another thing to worry about

- Try to eat oily fish twice a week

Food labelling

How do you choose healthy foods?

Food labelling can help you to make informed choices about whether to include a particular food in your diet. You can now choose from a wide selection of imported fresh foods with a long shelf-life. This is partly the result of improved storage methods such as refrigeration and freezing. Other ways to extend shelf-life are the addition of chemicals and the use of irradiation to delay spoiling. Before you buy food, you may wish to consider whether it has been treated to increase its acceptability and, if so, how safe these treatments are.

Food labelling laws

The Labelling of Food Regulations (1970) introduced criteria for claims about energy content, vitamins and minerals. By the mid-1980s, food manufacturers began using nutritional labelling as a marketing tool. This, and pressure from health professionals and consumers, led to further legislation in the Food Labelling Regulations (1996) (for more information, see www.food.gov.uk).

Extending the shelf-life of foods

Food-preserving techniques prevent the contamination and deterioration of food. They act by inhibiting bacterial activity and the action of enzymes in the foods that break down cells

Refrigeration
Reducing the storage temperature to 3 to 5°C reduces the deterioration of fats (rancidity) and slows down microbial growth

Freezing
Reducing the storage temperature to −18 to −20°C stops the growth of microbes but does not kill them. Microbes will still be present, and will resume growth once the food is defrosted. The deterioration of fats is slowed even further by freezing than by refrigeration, but will not stop if the food is defrosted. This is why food should not be refrozen after thawing

Chemicals
Altering the chemical composition of food reduces the impact of microbe contamination and oxidation

Irradiation
High doses of radiation sterilise food. Low doses can be used to delay ripening of fruit

The information on a food label?
Name
As well as the name of the food, all labels should list:

- ingredients

- date by which the food should be eaten

- storage instructions to prevent spoilage

- preparation instructions if necessary
- additives, with E numbers
- nutritional information
- genetically modified ingredients
- manufacturer details and batch number.

Names

Some foods have trade names, such as Frosted Flakes, whereas others have a descriptive name, such as gravy browning. Names such as wholemeal are defined by law. The name must be precise enough to distinguish the food from other products. There are exceptions for some foods, including whole, unpeeled fresh fruit and vegetables, flavourings, cheese and butter.

Names must not be misleading, for example, cherry cheesecake must have its flavour coming mainly from real cherries, as must a product with fresh cherries pictured on the packet. Cherry flavour, on the other hand, means that the product's flavour is derived mainly from artificial flavourings.

Ingredients

Most foods must have the ingredients listed in descending order of weight. Water is not always included, unless it falls within the constraints of legislation, because it is often considered an integral part of food. If added water takes up five per cent or more of the finished product, it must be listed with the other ingredients. There has been a recent trend towards listing water as aqua, presumably to make it sound less ordinary.

Food labels

By law, food labels must provide the consumer with specific kinds of information. These include the product name, ingredients (listed in descending order of weight) and details of the nutritional values.

Ingredients

Whole Wheat, Malt extract, Sugar, Salt, Colour: Annatto, Preservative: Sulphur Dioxide, Niacin, Iron, Riboflavin (B_2). Thiamine (B_1), Folic Acid

Nutritional information

	per 100g	per 37.5g serving
Energy	1440kJ	540kJ
	340kcal	128kcal
Protein	11.2g	4.2g
Carbohydrate	67.6g	25.4g
(of which sugars)	(4.7g)	(1.8g)
Fat	2.7g	1.0g
(of which saturates)	(0.6g)	(0.2g)
Fibre	10.5g	3.9g
Soluble	3.2g	1.3g
Insoluble	7.3g	2.7g
Sodium	0.4g	0.2g

Vitamins	per 100g	per 37.5g serving
Thiamine (B_1)	1.2mg/85% RDA	0.4mg/32% RDA
Riboflavin (B_2)	1.4mg/85% RDA	0.5mg/32% RDA
Niacin	15.3mg/85% RDA	5.7mg/32% RDA
Folic Acid	170.0µg/85% RDA	63.8µg/32% RDA
Iron	11.9mg/85% RDA	4.5mg/32% RDA

An average serving of 37.5g will provide 32% of the recommended daily allowance (RDA) for the average adult of the vitamins and iron listed

Made in England by Another plc

Best Before End: Nov 20

900g

Additives and E numbers

Ingredients that fall into this category are usually added in small quantities and therefore appear towards the end of the list. The approved name or E number may be used. An E number indicates that the additive is permitted under European Union legislation. Additives are used for flavouring, sweetening or colouring, to enhance the preservation of food or to affect its consistency or texture. Additives are discussed separately in 'Food additives' on page 98.

Date mark

Foods that have a shelf-life greater than three months must show a month and year by which they should be eaten. Foods with a shelf-life of less than three months must show the day and month by which they should be used. Products with a 'sell by' date rather than a 'best before' date should tell you within how many days the food should be eaten from this 'sell by' date. Retailers can be prosecuted for displaying products for sale after these dates.

Storage

Following storage instructions prevents food spoilage, reduces the risk of food poisoning and ensures that foods are eaten at their best. Star symbols are frequently shown to indicate a food's suitability for refrigeration or freezing.

Preparation

For foods that need heating, labels provide suitable information on temperature and timing for both conventional and microwave cookers, to ensure that food tastes at its best. Following cooking instructions ensures that food is thoroughly heated, reducing the risk of food poisoning.

Nutritional claims

Some of the terms used by manufacturers to describe their products are defined in law, to avoid the possibility that consumers may be misled, but others remain vague and undefined.

Claim	Meaning
Fat	
Low or reduced fat	25 per cent less fat than normal product
Fat free	Not more than 0.15 gram of fat per 100 grams
Virtually fat free	No legal definition
Energy*	
Reduced calorie	25 per cent less calories than normal product
Low calorie	Not more than 40 kcal per gram or millilitre
Diet, light or Lite	No legal definitions
Sugar**	
Sugar free	Not more than 0.2 gram per 100 grams
Reduced sugar	25 per cent less sugar than normal product
Salt (sodium)	
Reduced salt	25 per cent less salt than normal product or sodium
Low salt	Not more than 40 mg per serving (or 40 mg per 100 gram serving)
Salt free	Less than 5 mg per 100 grams

Nutritional claims (contd)

Claim	Meaning
Fibre	There is no legal definition of high fibre but many manufacturers use a level of at least 6 grams per 100 grams of food to mean high in fibre

*Manufacturers use the phrase 'as part of a low calorie diet' to imply that a particular product could be useful when on a slimming diet. Any food can be fitted into such a diet if other food and drink are adjusted to accommodate it. Some products are misleadingly labelled 'slimming' in that, weight for weight, they may have the same or even more calories than equivalent non-slimming foods, but because they are less dense (for example, some breakfast cereals) or are prepared in a particular way (for example, taken in water rather than milk), the energy per serving is lower.

**No added sugar also means no honey, fructose or fruit syrup. A list of names used for sugars in the manufacture of food is given in 'Carbohydrates' on page 47.

Ingredients that may cause allergies

Labels must state clearly if they contain ingredients to which people may be allergic or intolerant. It must be clear if any of these ingredients are present. For example, it is not enough to state 'glaze'; the label must state 'glaze made from eggs'. A list of such ingredients is shown on page 111.

Converting metric and imperial measures

Grams/ Kilograms	Ounces/ Pounds	Millilitres/ Litres	Pints
250 g	9 oz	250 ml	0.44
500 g	1 lb 2 oz	500 ml	0.88
750 g	1 lb 11 oz	750 ml	1.32
1 kg	2 lb 3 oz	1 litre	1.76
2 kg	4 lb 6 oz	2 litres	3.52
3 kg	6 lb 9 oz	4.54 litres	8 (1 gallon)

Nutritional claims

According to voluntary guidelines issued by the Food Standards Agency, nutritional values should be expressed per 100 grams of food, and per portion if the packet contains less than 100 grams. It is now a legal requirement for food weights to be in grams and kilograms, although some manufacturers quote both metric and imperial weights.

Information should be given about energy, protein, fat and carbohydrate, then about dietary fibre and sodium, and then about sugars, vitamins and minerals. Vitamin and mineral values are given when they are present in amounts greater than one-sixth of the recommended dietary intake.

Manufacturers who falsify claims can be prosecuted. However, the terminology used can be confusing. For example, 'low fat' has a legal definition, but 'lower in fat' can mean anything less than normal for that product category.

Genetically modified foods

Any ingredient that has been involved in gene modification, either human or animal genes, must appear on the label as dictated by the Genetically Modified and Novel Foods Regulations of England and Scotland.

Manufacturer and batch numbers

Manufacturers give their contact details on product labels, enabling consumers to write or telephone with enquiries or complaints, if necessary. All foods are marked with an identity number to allow both manufacturers and consumers to identify food batches easily.

Recommended daily allowance

Nutrition labelling often includes the recommended daily allowance (RDA) of energy, protein, vitamins or minerals. This is the amount that will supply the requirements of most people. There is no RDA for carbohydrate or fat because they are interchangeable sources of energy. A substance can only be listed in this way when more than one-sixth of the RDA is present.

The Government panel on the content of nutrients in the diet (Panel on Dietary Reference Values of the Committee on Medical Aspects of Food Policy, 1991) introduced two other terms: estimated average requirement (EAR) and reference nutrient intake (RNI). EAR is defined for energy, protein and vitamins for a specified group of people, for example, a specific age range. About half of this group will need more than the EAR and the other half will need less.

RNI, which is defined for protein, vitamins and minerals, is the amount that is enough for about 97 per cent of the population. For example, the EAR of women aged 19 to 50 years for riboflavin is 0.9 milligrams per day. The RNI is 1.1 milligrams per day. Most people will not need more than the EAR.

However, if the average intake of riboflavin is 1.1 milligrams per day or more, at least 97.5 per cent of the population will receive enough.

These data are included on food labels for information and as a marketing tool. In everyday life, such precise knowledge is not needed. If you and your family are eating a balanced diet following the guidelines in 'Healthy eating' on page 75, you are unlikely to be deficient in any nutrient.

Guideline daily amounts

Some food manufacturers give guideline daily amounts (GDAs) on packaging. GDAs summarise recommendations for energy, fat, sugar and salts and are intended as a guide when comparing products. Further details are available from the Institute of Grocery Distribution website (www.igd.com).

KEY POINTS

- Food labelling helps you to decide whether to buy food products, now that there is more storage, preserving and processing

- Laws determine what nutritional claims manufacturers may make

- The list of ingredients tells you what ingredients the food contains and in what proportions

- RDA is the recommended daily allowance that will supply the requirements of almost everyone

- Following manufacturers' guidelines for food storage and preparation can reduce the risk of food poisoning

Food additives

The debate over additives

Without additives, the variety of foods available and their shelf-lives would be greatly reduced. However, the use of additives in food is a controversial subject, with claims that they can trigger allergies or are toxic. Some people are sensitive to certain additives, especially colourings, and should check food labels carefully to see what additives the food contains.

Why use additives?

Many of the foods that we eat today contain additives. Additives are used in food for many reasons including the following:

- To keep foods fresh until eaten, widening food choice
- To enable food to be conveniently packaged, stored, prepared and used
- To make the product look more appealing
- To extend the food's shelf-life
- To reduce the ingredient cost
- To add additional nutrients

Approximately 3,500 additives are in use today. The Food Standards Agency is responsible for the control of additives and has a full list of them.

All permitted additives are considered safe and necessary, and are controlled by law. Food additives must gain approval before their use in food manufacture is permitted. Many additives are natural substances; for example, ascorbic acid (vitamin C) is used as a flour improver to speed up bread production. Natural additives must also undergo testing and approval before they can be used in food manufacture.

E numbers

E numbers are given to permitted food additives regarded as safe for use within the European Union. Some additives have a number but no E prefix, as they are under consideration for licensing by the EU. All food labels must show the additive's name or E number in the list of ingredients.

Colourings (E100–180)

Some examples of natural and synthetic colourings are shown on page 100. Food is coloured to restore losses that occur in manufacture and storage, to meet consumer expectations and to maintain uniformity of products. An example of this is that oranges have green patches when picked and are coloured orange before sale.

Preservatives (E200–290)

Food spoils easily: bacteria cause the structure to rot and putrefy; enzymes cause changes such as browning; injury causes some fruit cells to die, leading to discolouring and eventually rotting; fats become rancid as a result of oxidation. Preservatives stop food

Examples of natural and synthetic colourings

Many colours are used for cosmetic reasons. About half are natural pigments, such as carbon and riboflavin. Artificial colourings such as tartrazine and amaranth are also used.

Name	Colour	E number	Typical use
Natural colours			
Riboflavin	Yellow	E101	Processed cheese
Chlorophyll	Green	E140	Fats, oils, canned vegetables
Carbon	Black	E153	Jams and jellies
Alpha-carotene	Yellow/orange	E160	Margarine and cakes
Synthetic colours			
Tartrazine	Yellow	E102	Soft drinks
Sunset	Yellow	E110	Orange drinks
Amaranth	Red	E123	Blackcurrant products
Erythrosine	Red	E127	Glacé cherries
Indigo Carmine	Blue	E132	Savoury food mixes
Green S	Green	E142	Tinned peas, mint jelly and sauce

going off in these ways and make a wide range of goods available out of the usual season.

Traditional preservatives include salt, vinegar, alcohol and spices. Acetic acid is the major component of vinegar and may be considered as a natural additive, but it has undergone extensive testing and has an E number (E260).

Frequently used preservatives

Preservatives stop or prevent the growth of micro-organisms that can cause food poisoning. The most common preservatives added to processed foods include nitrates and sulphites.

Name	E number	Food use
Sorbic acid*	E200–E203	Cheese, yoghurt and soft drinks
Acetic acid	E260	Pickles and sauces
Lactic acid	E270	Margarine, confect-ionery and sauces
Propionic acid*	E280–E283	Bread, cakes and flour confectionery
Benzoic acid*	E210–E219	Soft drinks, pickles, fruit products
Sulphur dioxide	E220	Soft drinks, fruit products, beer, cider, wine
Nitrites	E249, E250	Cured meats, cooked meats and meat products
Nitrates	E251, E252	Bacon, ham and cheese (not Cheddar or Cheshire)

*Includes derivative products.

Radiation

Radiation can be used as a preservative because it destroys bacteria and enzymes that spoil food. It can also be used to delay ripening of fruit and sprouting in vegetables such as potatoes. This process is used only under licence and is monitored by a Government committee.

Other preservatives

Benzoic acid and benzoates

These preservatives are found in many fresh foods such as peas, bananas and berries. Benzoates cause adverse reactions in some people.

Sulphur dioxide

Sulphur dioxide is used as a preservative to destroy yeasts, which can cause fermentation in food products. Its use is not permitted in foods that are a significant source of the vitamin thiamine, because sulphur dioxide destroys thiamine.

Nitrates and nitrites

These preservatives kill bacteria that cause botulism, a potentially lethal form of food poisoning, and also preserve the red colour in meat. Nitrites may react with other chemicals in the gut to form nitrosamines, which have been shown to cause cancer in experimental animals, although there is no evidence that they do the same in people.

Antioxidants (E300–322)

Fats and oils become rancid through oxidation, which causes an unpleasant taste and smell. The higher the fat content of a product, the faster the food becomes

Permitted antioxidants

Antioxidants prevent or delay the effects of oils and fats turning food rancid. Some antioxidants are natural substances such as vitamins C and E. Others are synthetic, such as BHA and BHT.

Name	E number	Food use
Ascorbic acid (vitamin C)*	E300–E305	Beer, soft drinks, powdered milk, fruit and meat products
Tocopherols (vitamin E)*	E306–E309	Vegetable oils
Gallates	E310–E320	Vegetable oils and fats, margarine
Butylated hydroxyanisole (BHA)	E320	Margarine and fat in baked products, e.g. pies
Butylated hydroxytoluene (BHT)	E321	Crisps, margarine, vegetable oils and fats, convenience foods

*Includes derivative products.

rancid. This process can be delayed, but not stopped, by low temperatures (for example, refrigeration). The use of antioxidants prevents oxidation.

The most common antioxidants are butylated hydroxyanisole (BHA) and butylated hydroxytoluene (BHT).

Emulsifiers and stabilisers (E400–495)

These additives are used to increase the shelf-life of foods and affect their texture and consistency. Emulsifiers are fatty compounds that change the chemical properties of some foods so that they can be mixed. An example of this is vinaigrette, which will normally separate out with oil floating on the top of the vinegar. If an emulsifier, such as lecithin, is added, the oil and vinegar stay mixed together in an emulsion.

Examples of emulsifiers and stabilisers

Emulsifiers are used to prevent the oil and water components of many foods from separating. Stabilisers are added to improve texture and are often made from plant matter such as seaweed.

Name	E number	Food use	Category
Lecithins*	E322	Chocolate, margarine and potato snacks	Emulsifier
Citric acid**	E472a–c	Pickles, dairy and baked products	"
Tartaric acid**	E472d–f	Baking powder	"
Alginic acid**	E400–E401	Ice cream, instant desserts and puddings	"
Agar	E406	Tinned ham, ice cream	"
Carrageenan	E407	Ice cream	"
Gums	E410–E415	Ice cream, soups and confectionery	"
Pectin	E440	Preserves and jellies	Stabiliser

*May also be used as an antioxidant.
**Includes derivative products.

Stabilisers (for example, pectin) are usually large carbohydrates. They form a structure that is capable of holding the smaller chemicals in foods together, forming a more stable product. This is the largest group of additives and many are natural substances – for example, carrageenan, which is derived from seaweed and is used as a gelling agent.

Thickeners are carbohydrates that alter or control the consistency of a product during cooling or heating, or in storage.

Raising agents are used to give a light spongy texture to cakes and other baked products, and include bicarbonate of soda, tartaric acid and baking powder (a mixture of sodium bicarbonate and sodium pyrophosphoric acid).

Sweeteners

These are divided into two groups. Caloric sweeteners add energy to the diet, and include mannitol, sorbitol, xylitol and hydrogenated glucose syrup. Non-caloric sweeteners are synthetic sweeteners, and include acesulfame K, aspartame, saccharin and thaumatin. Sucrose, glucose, fructose and lactose are all classified as foods rather than sweeteners or additives.

Fortifiers

Foods can be fortified to reduce the risk of deficiency diseases within a population. Fortification takes place either when a particular nutrient has been lost during processing, or when the addition of a nutrient(s) is beneficial to health. By law, flour is fortified with certain B vitamins, calcium and iron, and margarine is fortified with vitamins A and D. Voluntary fortification includes the addition of B vitamins and iron to breakfast cereals and infant formulas. Vegan products are sometimes fortified with vitamin B_{12}.

Other additives

Glazing agents are used to give food an appealing shiny appearance, and include egg-based products. Flour improvers are used to produce bread with a lighter texture and to slow staling.

Other additives include: flavour enhancers, such as monosodium glutamate (which intensifies the flavour of food); anti-foaming agents (which prevent frothing during processing); and propellant gases (which are used, for example, in aerosol cream). Polyphosphates enable products to retain water, so increasing their weight, and are used in foods such as frozen poultry and cured meats.

KEY POINTS

■ Food additives prolong the shelf-life of foods and make them more appealing to eat

■ If you are concerned about the safety of additives, check food labels carefully

■ Fortified foods supplement dietary intakes of certain nutrients

Food allergy and intolerance

What is a food allergy?

Food allergies and intolerances cause similar symptoms, but involve different mechanisms.

Food allergies are caused by the immune system reacting abnormally to food. Most food could trigger an allergic response, but preparation, cooking and the action of digestive acid and enzymes destroy most of this potential.

When your body's defence system meets a potentially harmful substance, it responds with an immunological reaction. This releases histamine and other chemicals into your circulation, causing itching of the skin and changes in blood vessels. In serious cases, the changes in blood vessels can lead to a rapid fall in blood volume and a dramatic, and potentially fatal, reaction, known as anaphylactic shock, which can interfere with a person's ability to breathe. The chemicals released in this reaction also cause constriction of lung tissues and are associated with asthma.

What is a food intolerance?

Food intolerances do not involve an immunological reaction. Some of the mechanisms involved are not fully understood. Food intolerance reactions include the following.

Non-allergic histamine release

Shellfish and strawberries cause this reaction in some people, who usually develop a rash.

Enzyme defects

People with a lactase deficiency, for example, have a reduced ability to digest the milk sugar lactose. The treatment consists of a diet low in milk and milk products.

Pharmacological reactions

These occur in response to food components, such as amines. Amines are found in foods that contain nitrogen (for example, amino acids in foods such as tea, coffee, cola drinks and chocolate). The effects may

Lactose intolerance

People with lactose deficiency should avoid the products listed below. Several lactose-reduced milks and products are available commercially.

- Cows', goats' and sheep's milk
- Milk products, such as cheese and skimmed milk
- Milk derivatives often used in food manufacture. Remember to read the list of ingredients
- Foods such as stock cubes and crisps, which often contain whey
- Medicines that use milk products as fillers

be triggered by small amounts of food and include migraine, tremor, sweating and palpitations, which can be alarming.

Irritant effects
Foods such as curry can irritate the gut. Monosodium glutamate can cause a condition known as Chinese restaurant syndrome, which results in chest pain, palpitations and weakness.

Diagnosing an allergy
Anyone suspected of having a food allergy must be diagnosed and treated by a dietitian. Diagnosis often involves eliminating possible allergens – substances that cause an allergic reaction – from the diet. An elimination diet is sometimes based on the very few foods that are unlikely to cause allergic reactions, and such a limited diet is difficult to plan and stick to. As each food is gradually reintroduced to the diet, the dietitian can assess which of them is responsible for any symptoms.

This process needs careful monitoring. It is not safe to try excluding suspect foods from your diet by yourself. If it is necessary to use a very restrictive diet, there is a risk of nutritional deficiencies developing, unless it is carefully controlled. This is especially important in children, who need an adequate supply of the right nutrients in order to grow normally and maintain good health.

The danger of anaphylaxis, or other severe reactions associated with the diagnosis of food allergy, means that the dietitian works closely with medical colleagues.

Foods that may cause allergies

Manufacturers must show clearly the presence of the following in any product, as they may cause allergies:

- Celery
- Cereals containing gluten: wheat, rye, oats, barley
- Crustaceans, for example lobster, crab
- Milk
- Eggs
- Fish
- Mustard
- Soybeans
- Peanuts
- Nuts: almonds, pistachios, brazil nuts, walnuts, hazelnuts, cashews, pecans, macadamia nuts
- Sesame seeds
- Sulphur dioxide and sulphites at levels above 10 milligrams per kilogram or litre.

Preventing food allergies

Many people do themselves more harm then good by excluding nutritionally important foods (such as milk), to which they believe they have an allergy. Get expert advice before following this course. Some food allergies are inherited or may be related to a child becoming sensitised while in the womb or in the first months after birth.

Atopic eczema

Atopic eczema affects children with a family history of allergies, including hay fever and asthma, and has been linked to food allergies. Some people have suggested that pregnant and breast-feeding women should change their diets to reduce or prevent the risk of their children developing allergies to foods.

Mothers of children at risk of developing atopic eczema (the kind that runs in families, often together with asthma) should try to avoid highly allergenic foods such as milk and milk products, nuts, eggs and soya beans. It may also be worth delaying the introduction of any of these foods to the children until they are over eight months old. Breast milk appears to give some protection, but no one is sure whether cows' milk plays any role in triggering allergies. Despite an increase in breast-feeding in the UK, atopic eczema is more common than it used to be.

Nut allergy

Peanuts are the most common cause of the serious (and sometimes fatal) allergic reaction known as anaphylaxis. Immediate medical attention is usually needed, although some people who are aware of their allergy carry medication to counteract their body's response. Not all peanut allergy sufferers have such a dramatic and rapid allergic reaction.

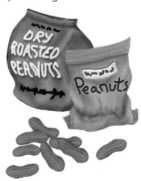

Recent studies have shown that peanut allergy is more common than previously realised and appears to be on the increase. This is probably related to the fact that women often eat larger quantities of peanuts and products containing peanut oil while pregnant or breast-feeding. Peanut and other nut allergies can be inherited, and any women with a family history of this type of allergy should avoid these foods during pregnancy and breast-feeding.

Hyperactivity

A link between hyperactive children and food additives was first suggested in the 1970s. Some scientists have found that the behaviour of these children improve when certain foods are eliminated from their diet. These include milk, eggs, wheat, nuts and colourings and preservatives such as tartrazine and benzoic acid. There is a link between food and hyperactivity in a minority of children, especially those with allergic conditions such as asthma and eczema. However, there is no conclusive evidence that any food is responsible for triggering the behaviour of most hyperactive children.

Case study: coeliac disease

Margaret was experiencing tiredness, weight loss, abdominal pain and diarrhoea, with bulky, foul-smelling stools that were difficult to flush away. Blood tests showed that she was anaemic, with iron and folate deficiencies. A tissue sample taken from her jejunum (small intestine) showed that her intestinal wall was flat with few of the characteristic projections called villi.

Margaret had a condition called coeliac disease. The wall of her jejunum was reacting to gluten, a constituent of wheat, as if it was toxic. Gluten makes wheat products such as cake and bread rise. The flattening of the villi meant that Margaret was unable to absorb nutrients properly, resulting in weight loss and deficiencies, causing anaemia and diarrhoea. The bulky, offensive stools were caused by a failure to absorb fat properly. They were difficult to flush away because of their high fat content.

Margaret's doctor prescribed iron and folate supplements to cure the anaemia and referred her to a dietitian specialising in gastrointestinal problems. She began a gluten-free diet, avoiding all products containing wheat, rye and barley. The dietitian told Margaret that not everyone agrees with the need to avoid oats, but suggested that she do so to begin with. Later, she could put them back on the menu to see whether her symptoms then recurred.

A gluten-free diet is not easy to follow, because products such as flour are included in many food products as a thickening agent. Even small quantities of gluten may cause trouble to coeliac patients. Margaret found that it was essential to read food labels and obtained gluten-free food lists from Coeliac UK. Her GP was able to prescribe gluten-free products.

Margaret's symptoms took several months to improve. She will have to remain on the diet for life to get permanent relief from her symptoms.

Case study: lactose intolerance

Ken was admitted to a specialist nutrition unit because he was seriously obese. He was assessed to see whether he was suitable for a controversial treatment that involved wiring his jaw so that his mouth could open only very slightly.

Ken had never particularly liked milk, but was resigned to the fact that, if he did have his jaws wired, it would become a major component of his diet. It was decided to go ahead with the treatment. Under medical supervision, Ken started a diet based on full-fat milk. Shortly afterwards, he developed nausea, bloating, abdominal pain and diarrhoea. It was discovered that Ken was intolerant to the milk sugar lactose. The dietitian devised another diet for Ken based on fermented milk products, such as yoghurt.

KEY POINTS

- Food allergies involve immunological reactions; food intolerances involve many different non-immunological mechanisms

- Never put your child on a restricted diet, even if you suspect an allergy, without getting expert advice first, no matter how mild the symptoms

Dietary supplements, alternative diets and 'health foods'

A growing range

The growing interest in diet and health has stimulated an increase in the market for dietary supplements. The range of supplements available in health food shops, chemists and supermarkets is growing, with vitamins, minerals, fish liver oils and evening primrose oil being the most popular.

Dietary supplements fall between medicines and foods in terms of legal controls, and it is therefore difficult to regulate the way that they are promoted and sold. Some manufacturers make misleading claims about what their products can do and provide little, if any, information on possible side effects and the hazards of overdosing. No medical claims can legally be made for these products unless they have been thoroughly tested and licensed.

Nutrient supplements

The role of vitamins and minerals is well established (see 'Vitamins and minerals' on page 62). However, the use of large doses is controversial. Most people living in the UK shouldn't need to take supplements to avoid becoming deficient in vitamins or minerals. A balanced diet will provide nutrients in sufficient quantities to satisfy your body's requirements.

The only people who need supplements are those who have medical conditions affecting the absorption or metabolism of certain nutrients and those who have increased needs. Housebound elderly people may require vitamin D supplements. Their limited exposure to sunlight reduces the amount of vitamin D that they can synthesise.

Folate and iron

The need to supplement the diet of pregnant women with folate and iron is one of the few exceptions. Folate supplementation before conception and in early pregnancy has been shown to reduce the incidence of neural tube defects such as spina bifida. The need to take iron in pregnancy is not totally accepted by doctors; some argue that the low blood concentrations of iron are due to a normal dilution by the increased blood volume that occurs in pregnancy. The amount of iron normally taken by pregnant women does not, however, appear to cause side effects so, although it may not always do any good, it does no harm either.

Pyridoxine

Many other supplements make claims that have little or no scientific justification. Pyridoxine supplements are taken by many women to reduce symptoms associated with premenstrual syndrome, although there is no conclusive evidence to show that they work. Some research studies have shown that daily doses of 500 milligrams or more over several months may damage nerves in the feet and hands.

Vitamins for children

There is no evidence to support the theory that giving children vitamin supplements makes them more intelligent. All children need a balanced diet to function normally and to grow, and any dietary problems will obviously undermine their ability to do their school work well.

The Consumers Association

The Consumers Association supports EU legislation on food supplements, which came into effect in 2005. The legislation sets safety and quality standards for supplements. For example, there are regulations about the chemical form that the vitamins and minerals are in and about the minimum levels of vitamins and minerals that a supplement must include. The following must be shown on the label:

- details of the nutrients included
- the amount recommended to be taken daily
- a warning not to exceed this dose
- a statement that supplements should not be used as a substitute for a varied diet
- a warning to keep the product out of reach of children.

High-energy and protein supplements

These products are aimed at exercise enthusiasts who want to eat more calories as they use up more energy. These people are often trying to increase their muscle mass and require more protein to do this. Calories are used mainly by lean tissue, of which muscle is a major component. As the muscle mass increases, more calories are needed to maintain the more muscular frame. These extra calories and protein can easily be supplied by eating more food.

Elderly convalescents and their carers may also use these supplements. The products are often based on milk and need to be mixed with milk before they are used. Although they may be of some benefit, their strong flavourings and rich nature make them unpalatable to some people with poor appetites. It is usually better to offer convalescents frequent, small snacks and meals consisting of foods that they like and therefore will eat.

'Health foods'

This term is usually used to describe foods that are not readily available in supermarkets but which are sold in specialist shops. The name implies that these foods are particularly healthy. This is misleading, as people who already eat a balanced diet are unlikely to derive any benefit from them. However, there are many useful products sold in health food shops. Wholemeal foods are a good example, although you can normally buy them just as easily in your local supermarket.

Organic foods such as cereals, fruit and vegetables are becoming more widely available in both specialist shops and supermarkets, but they are invariably more expensive as a result of higher production costs. The use of natural farming methods has obvious advantages in reducing the reliance on pesticides and fertilisers. However, there is little scientific evidence to support the theory that organic foods are healthier than those produced by modern methods.

Functional foods

Over the last few years a new type of food has lined supermarket and health shop shelves. These foods are known as functional foods and are fortified with a range of phytochemicals that suggest that they can treat or prevent certain diseases such as heart disease. Any product should be assessed by its individual merits, but it is important to remember that nothing can replace the benefits of a healthy balanced diet.

Phyto-oestrogens are a group of compounds found naturally in plant foods. The best food sources are soyabean and its products such as textured vegetable protein, tofu, tempeh and soya milk/flour. Recently, there has been interest in the role of phyto-oestrogens in the relief of menopausal symptoms, such as hot flushes. Although phyto-oestrogens appear to be a natural alternative to HRT, there is only limited research to support this at present.

Foods containing bacteria

In adults the gastrointestinal tract contains about one kilogram and 500 different types of bacteria. The presence and balance of these bacteria are important and, if this balance is disturbed, the health of the gastrointestinal tract will be affected. Recently, products have become available that help to maintain this balance. Probiotics contain live bacteria – for example, lactobacilli – which help prevent disease in the gut. There is some evidence to suggest that they reduce the incidence of diarrhoea and may help lactose intolerance. Manufacturers must, however, fulfil strict criteria about their safety, production and storage.

Bacteria in the gut require substances to help them grow and prebiotics – for example, fructo-oligosaccharides – are products that do this. They help the beneficial bacteria to grow and may therefore be useful in the treatment of constipation. Prebiotics are found in a range of foods, including dairy and bakery products. Both probiotics and prebiotics are being investigated further to look at their potential benefits.

Alternative diets

In modern society, health is a major concern, and people are always looking to optimise the benefits from their diet. At times, this has resulted in an increase in the number of people willing to pay for alternative diets, many of which are expensive with debatable, if any, benefits.

Detoxification diets

These are recommended by various health writers and therapists to cleanse the body, and often involve fasting, bathing and exfoliating (removal of dead skin by rubbing and brushing) to remove toxins. If your liver and kidneys are functioning properly, your body will clear any waste substances naturally. There is no scientific evidence to support the benefits of these diets. Always consult your medical practitioner before trying one of them.

Anti-candida diets

It has been suggested that overgrowth of yeasts, particularly *Candida albicans*, can lead to a variety of debilitating symptoms. This overgrowth is supposedly triggered by diets rich in yeasts and sugar (which is used as food by yeasts), oral contraceptives and the use of broad-spectrum antibiotics. This is alleged to result in toxin production, which weakens the immune system, making susceptible people prone to a wide range of illnesses. The diet used to treat this condition involves avoiding bread, vinegar, alcohol, pickles, cheese, yeast extracts and all products containing sucrose. There is no medically controlled evidence to justify the use of these diets.

Food-combining (Hay) diet

Supporters of diets such as this claim that the body cannot digest acid and alkaline foods together. They also claim that mixing protein and carbohydrate foods results in many health problems, such as headaches, allergies and obesity. In reality, the digestive system is fully capable of digesting a meal containing a mixture of foods, using varying acid and alkaline conditions.

Slimming diets

There are many diets that are supposed to make it easy for people to lose weight. Many totally eliminate one food group from the diet. It is suggested that these diets 'burn fat' or 'speed up the metabolism'. Some slimming diets are based on single foods, such as grapefruit. Such claims have no scientific basis and, if you succeed in losing weight on these diets, it is because of their restrictive nature. Such diets will not help you change to a healthy eating pattern in the long term. They can also cause nutritional deficiencies.

Very-low-calorie diets

Very-low-calorie diets (VLCDs) were very popular in the 1980s and provided less than 400 kcal per day. Medical evidence linked these diets to cardiac problems. A Government committee recommended that these diets should not be used for longer than three to four weeks and then only by obese people under medical supervision. The energy content and presentation of these diets were then changed to provide 600 to 800 kcal per day, incorporating snack bars and prepared meals. Their popularity has greatly declined over recent years.

The Atkins diet

Low-carbohydrate diets, for example, the Atkins diet, were first promoted in the 1960s but have recently become very popular. Reducing your intake of carbohydrate leads to the mobilisation of fat stores, releasing chemicals called ketones. Ketones are made from the breakdown of fat and can be used by the body, but not the brain, as an energy source for a limited period. These diets succeed in restricting energy intake, as many people find it difficult to eat large amounts of fat or protein without carbohydrate. The lack of carbohydrate results in the rapid use of glycogen energy stores and this also causes the loss of water, which accounts for the initial rapid weight loss. When carbohydrate is reintroduced into the diet, weight gain occurs.

The healthiest approach

The best approach to losing weight is to adopt a healthy diet. This will make sure that your weight remains as it should be in the long term, as well as providing all the nutrients you need for good health (see 'Healthy eating' on page 75).

Case study: loss of appetite

At 74, Sophie was becoming frail. She had recently had major surgery and was staying with her daughter, Hilary, to convalesce. Hilary and her family were health conscious and had a varied, balanced, high-fibre, low-fat diet. She used a lot of wholemeal products, especially pasta and granary breads. Hilary believed that this diet would speed up her mother's recovery.

Unfortunately, Sophie's appetite was poor and she was becoming increasingly uninterested in food. She didn't like pasta, preferring more 'traditional' meals. The district nurse advised Hilary to talk to the dietitian at the local health centre. She gave Hilary advice on ways to encourage Sophie to eat more, and recommended giving Sophie meals that she would eat and enjoy rather than providing 'healthy' foods.

The dietitian advised Hilary to follow a few simple guidelines:

- Remember that high-energy supplements can be over-whelming and very filling. Milky drinks are often a more acceptable alternative.

- Give plenty of fluids, but not immediately before a meal as they may reduce the appetite.

- Ask Sophie's doctor whether vitamin supplements would be helpful; some prescribed drugs can interact with nutrients in the diet or affect absorption.

- Take care when reducing fat in her diet as this may affect her vitamin D and calcium levels.

Hilary began providing smaller meals of simple dishes that Sophie liked more than pasta and granary bread. A supplement that they found useful was a hot chocolate drink made with Complan before bed. Once

Sophie's appetite had returned, Hilary was able to increase the portions so that her mother gradually gained weight.

KEY POINTS

- The use of specialised food supplements is often unnecessary

- Normal foods can be modified to provide any additional requirements

- Lack of appetite is an important factor when trying to persuade someone to eat more

- Most healthy people are unlikely to experience any specific nutrient deficiency

Useful information

We have included the following organisations because, on preliminary investigation, they may be of use to the reader. However, we do not have first-hand experience of each organisation and so cannot guarantee the organisation's integrity. The reader must therefore exercise his or her own discretion and judgement when making further enquiries.

Allergy UK
3 White Oak Square, London Road
Swanley
Kent BR8 7AG
Tel: 01322 619898
Fax: 01322 663480
Helpline: 020 8303 8583
Email: info@allergyuk.org
Website: www.allergyuk.org

Offers information on all types of allergies, quarterly newsletter and support network; translation cards for travel abroad.

Ashwell Associates
Ashwell Street

Ashwell, Herts SG7 5PZ
Email:margaret@ashwell.uk.com
Website: www.ashwell.uk.com

Independent scientific consultants and disseminators of information on nutrition and food labelling. Shape chart available online to calculate disease risk based on waist circumference.

Asthma UK

England, Wales and N. Ireland
Summit House, 70 Wilson Street
London EC2A 2DB
Tel: 020 7786 4900
Fax: 020 7256 6075
Email: info@asthma.org.uk
Helpline: 0845 701 0203
Website: www.asthma.org.uk

Provides a wide range of information for people with asthma and their families. Helpline staffed by specialist asthma nurses. Has some support groups and funds medical research. Offers supervised holidays for young people with asthma.

Asthma UK, Scotland

4 Queen Street
Edinburgh EH2 1JE
Tel: 0131 226 2544
Fax: 0131 226 2401
Email: enquiries@asthma.org.uk
Helpline: 08457 010203
Website: www.asthma.org.uk

Provides a wide range of information for people with asthma and their families. Funds medical research.

Benefits Enquiry Line
Helpline: 0800 882200
Website: www.dwp.gov.uk
Minicom: 0800 243355
N. Ireland: 0800 220674

Government agency giving information and advice on sickness and disability benefits for people with disabilities and their carers.

British Heart Foundation
14 Fitzhardinge Street
London W1H 6DH
Tel: 020 7935 0185
Fax: 020 7486 5820
Helpline: 0845 070 8070
Website: www.bhf.org.uk

Funds research, promotes education and raises money to buy equipment to treat heart disease. Information and support available for people with heart conditions. Via Heartstart UK, arranges training in emergency life-saving techniques for lay people.

British Nutrition Foundation
High Holborn House, 52–54 High Holborn
London WC1V 6RQ
Tel: 020 7404 6504
Fax: 020 7404 6747
Email: postbox@nutrition.org.uk
Website: www.nutrition.org.uk

Professional association that determines the scientific consensus in nutrition and communicates this through its free publications. An SAE requested for information as no telephone advice is available.

Coeliac UK

Suites A–D, Octagon Court
High Wycombe, Bucks HP11 2HS
Tel: 01494 437278
Fax: 01494 474349
Email: helpline@coeliac.co.uk
Helpline: 0870 444 8804
Website: www.coeliac.co.uk

Provides information and support for people medically diagnosed with coeliac disease and dermatitis herpetiformis.

Dairy Council

Henrietta House, 17–18 Henrietta Street
Covent Garden
London WC2E 8QH
Tel: 020 7395 4030
Fax: 020 7240 9679
Email: info@dairycouncil.org.uk
Website: www.milk.co.uk

Funded by the dairy industry to promote milk and dairy products.

Department for Environment, Food and Rural Affairs (DEFRA)

Nobel House, 17 Smith Square
London SW1P 3JR

Tel: 020 7238 6000
Fax: 020 7238 3329
Email: helpline@defra.gsi.gov.uk
Helpline: 08459 335577
Website: www.defra.gov.uk

Provides wide ranging information covering the environment, food and rural affairs.

Department of Health (DH)
PO Box 77
London SE1 6XH
Tel: 020 7210 4850
Fax: 01623 724524
Email: doh@prolog.uk.com
Helpline: 0800 555777
Website: www.doh.gov.uk/publications

Produces and distributes literature about general health matters.

Diabetes UK
Macleod House, 10 Parkway
London NW1 7AA
Tel: 020 7424 1000
Fax: 020 7424 1001
Helpline: 0845 120 2960
Textline: 020 7424 1888
Email: info@diabetes.org.uk
Website: www.diabetes.org.uk

Provides advice and information for people with diabetes and their families. Has local support groups.

CORE (Digestive Disorders Foundation)

3 St Andrew's Place, Regents Park
London NW1 4LB
Tel: 020 7486 0341
Fax: 020 7224 2012
Email: info@corecharity.org.uk
Website: www.corecharity.org.uk

Provides a range of information about the cause,
symptoms and treatment of digestive disorders. SAE
requested.

Food Standards Agency

Aviation House, 125 Kingsway
London WC2B 6NH
Tel: 020 7276 8000
Fax: 020 7238 6330
Website: www.eatwell.gov.uk

Advice on diet and health. Wide-ranging information
on additives, contaminants and chemical safety:
Additives: 020 7276 8570
Allergies and intolerance: 020 7276 8516
Contaminants: 020 7276 8713
Novel foods: 020 7276 8595
Chemical safety: 020 7276 8527

Heart UK

7 North Road
Maidenhead SL6 1PE
Tel: 01628 628638
Fax: 01628 628698
Email: ask@heartuk.org.uk
Website: www.heartuk.org.uk

Offers information, advice and support to people with coronary heart disease and especially those at high risk of familial hypercholesterolaemia. Members receive bimonthly magazine.

Hyperactive Children's Support Group, Dept W

71 Whyke Lane
Chichester, West Sussex PO19 7PD
Tel: 01243 539966
Fax: 01243 552019
Email: hyperactive@hacsg.org.uk
Website: www.hacsg.org.uk

Provides information and support, particularly with the dietary and nutritional aspects, for parents with a hyperactive child. For information, SAE requested.

NHS Direct

Tel: 0845 4647 (24 hours, 365 days a year)
Textphone: 0845 606 4647
Website: www.nhsdirect.nhs.uk
NHS Scotland: 0800 224488

Offers confidential health-care advice, information and referral service. A good first port of call for any health advice.

NHS Smoking Helpline

Tel: 0800 169 0169 (7am–11pm, 365 days a year)
Pregnancy smoking helpline: 0800 169 9169
(12 noon–9pm, 365 days a year)
Website: www.givingupsmoking.co.uk

Has advice, help and encouragement on giving up smoking. Specialist advisers available to offer on-going support to those who genuinely are trying to give up smoking. Can refer to local branches.

National Institute for Health and Clinical Excellence (NICE)

MidCity Place, 71 High Holborn
London WC1V 6NA
Tel: 020 7067 5800
Fax: 020 7067 5801
Email: nice@nice.nhs.uk
Website: www.nice.org.uk

Provides national guidance on the promotion of good health and the prevention and treatment of ill-health. Patient information leaflets are available for each piece of guidance issued.

Prodigy Website

Sowerby Centre for Health Informatics at Newcastle (SCHIN), Bede House, All Saints Business Centre
Newcastle upon Tyne NE1 2ES
Tel: 0191 2436100
Fax: 0191 2436101
Email: prodigy-enquiries@schin.co.uk
Website: www.prodigy.nhs.uk

A website mainly for GPs giving information for patients listed by disease plus named self-help organisations.

Quit (Smoking Quitlines)
211 Old Street
London EC1V 9NR
Tel: 020 7251 1551
Fax: 020 7251 1661
Helpline: 800 002200 (9am–9pm, 365 days a year)
Email: info@quit.org.uk
Website:www.quit.org.uk
Scotland: 0800 848484
Wales: 0800 169 0169 (NHS)

Offers individual advice on giving up smoking in
English and Asian languages. Talks to schools on
smoking and pregnancy and can refer to local support
groups. Runs training courses for professionals.

Vegan Society
Donald Watson House, 7 Battle Road
St Leonards-on-Sea, East Sussex TN37 7AA
Tel: 01424 427393
Fax: 01424 717064
Helpline: 08454 588244
Email: info@vegansociety.com
Website: www.vegansociety.com

Promotes a lifestyle that, as far as possible, excludes all
forms of exploitation of animals for food, clothing or
any other purpose. For an information pack, send two
first-class stamps or a large SAE.

Vegetarian Society
Parkdale, Dunham Road
Altrincham, Cheshire WA14 4QG
Tel: 0161 925 2000 (Mon–Fri 8.30am–5pm)

Fax: 0161 926 9182
Email: info@vegsoc.org
Website: www.vegsoc.org

Provides a starter pack on the vegetarian way of life and information sheet about fats and cholesterol. Send an A5 SAE for a list of local groups and cookery books.

Website

www.igd.com
Institute of Grocery Distribution

Information about guideline daily amounts (GDAs).

The internet as a further source of information

After reading this book, you may feel that you would like further information on the subject. The internet is of course an excellent place to look and there are many websites with useful information about medical disorders, related charities and support groups.

For those who do not have a computer at home some bars and cafes offer facilities for accessing the internet. These are listed in the Yellow Pages under 'Internet Bars and Cafes' and 'Internet Providers'. Your local library offers a similar facility and has staff to help you find the information that you need.

It should always be remembered, however, that the internet is unregulated and anyone is free to set up a website and add information to it. Many websites offer impartial advice and information that has been compiled and checked by qualified medical professionals. Some, on the other hand, are run by commercial organisations with the purpose of promoting their own products. Others still are run by pressure groups, some of which will provide carefully assessed and accurate information whereas others may be suggesting medications or treatments that are not supported by the medical and scientific community.

Unless you know the address of the website you want to visit – for example, www.familydoctor.co.uk – you may find the following guidelines useful when searching the internet for information.

Search engines and other searchable sites

Google (www.google.co.uk) is the most popular search engine used in the UK, followed by Yahoo! (http://uk.yahoo.com) and MSN (www.msn.co.uk). Also popular are the search engines provided by Internet Service Providers such as Tiscali and other sites such as the BBC site (www.bbc.co.uk).

In addition to the search engines that index the whole web, there are also medical sites with search facilities, which act almost like mini-search engines, but cover only medical topics or even a particular area of medicine. Again, it is wise to look at who is responsible for compiling the information offered to ensure that it is impartial and medically accurate. The NHS Direct site (www.nhsdirect.nhs.uk) is an example of a searchable medical site.

Links to many British medical charities can be found at the Association of Medical Charities website (www.amrc.org.uk) and at Charity Choice (www.charitychoice.co.uk).

Search phrases

Be specific when entering a search phrase. Searching for information on 'cancer' will return results for many different types of cancer as well as on cancer in general. You may even find sites offering astrological information. More useful results will be returned by using search phrases such as 'lung cancer' and 'treatments for lung cancer'. Both Google and Yahoo! offer an advanced search option that includes the ability to search for the exact phrase, enclosing the search phrase in quotes, that is, 'treatments for lung cancer' will have the same effect. Limiting a search to an exact phrase reduces the number of results returned but it is best to refine a search to an exact match only if you are not getting useful results with a normal search. Adding 'UK' to your search term will bring up mainly British sites, so a good phrase might be 'lung cancer' UK (don't include UK within the quotes).

Always remember the internet is international and unregulated. It holds a wealth of valuable information but individual sites may be biased, out of date or just plain wrong. Family Doctor Publications accepts no responsibility for the content of links published in this series.

Index

Your pages

We have included the following pages because they may help you manage your illness or condition and its treatment.

Before an appointment with a health professional, it can be useful to write down a short list of questions of things that you do not understand, so that you can make sure that you do not forget anything.

Some of the sections may not be relevant to your circumstances.

We are always pleased to receive constructive criticism or suggestions about how to improve the books. You can contact us at:

Email: familydoctor@btinternet.com
Letter: Family Doctor Publications
        PO Box 4664
        Poole
        BH15 1NN

Thank you

Health-care contact details

Name:

Job title:

Place of work:

Tel:

Name:

Job title:

Place of work:

Tel:

Name:

Job title:

Place of work:

Tel:

Name:

Job title:

Place of work:

Tel:

Significant past health events – illnesses/ operations/investigations/treatments

Event	Month	Year	Age (at time)

Appointments for health care

Name:

Place:

Date:

Time:

Tel:

Name:

Place:

Date:

Time:

Tel:

Name:

Place:

Date:

Time:

Tel:

Name:

Place:

Date:

Time:

Tel:

Appointments for health care

Name:

Place:

Date:

Time:

Tel:

Name:

Place:

Date:

Time:

Tel:

Name:

Place:

Date:

Time:

Tel:

Name:

Place:

Date:

Time:

Tel:

Current medication(s) prescribed by your doctor

Medicine name:

Purpose:

Frequency & dose:

Start date:

End date:

Medicine name:

Purpose:

Frequency & dose:

Start date:

End date:

Medicine name:

Purpose:

Frequency & dose:

Start date:

End date:

Medicine name:

Purpose:

Frequency & dose:

Start date:

End date:

Other medicines/supplements you are taking, not prescribed by your doctor

Medicine/treatment:

Purpose:

Frequency & dose:

Start date:

End date:

Medicine/treatment:

Purpose:

Frequency & dose:

Start date:

End date:

Medicine/treatment:

Purpose:

Frequency & dose:

Start date:

End date:

Medicine/treatment:

Purpose:

Frequency & dose:

Start date:

End date:

Questions to ask at appointments
(Note: do bear in mind that doctors work under great time pressure, so long lists may not be helpful for either of you)

Questions to ask at appointments
(Note: do bear in mind that doctors work under great time pressure, so long lists may not be helpful for either of you)

Notes

Notes

Notes